Ligament Balancing In Total Knee Arthroplasty

An Instructional Manual

Springer

Berlin
Heidelberg
New York
Hongkong
London
Milan
Paris
Tokyo

LEO A. WHITESIDE

Ligament Balancing in Total Knee Arthroplasty

An Instructional Manual

With 193 Figures

Springer

Leo A. Whiteside, M.D.
Missouri Bone and Joint Center
Biomechanical Research Laboratory
14825 Sugarwood Trail
St. Louis, MO 63014
USA

ISBN-13:978-3-642-63924-1 Springer-Verlag Berlin Heidelberg New York
Cataloging-in-Publication Date applied for
Ligament Balancing in Total Knee Arthroplasty – An Instructional Manual, L.A. Whiteside
Berlin; Heidelberg; New York; Hong Kong; London; Milan; Paris; Tokyo; Springer, 2004
ISBN-13:978-3-642-63924-1 e-ISBN-13:978-3-642-59295-9
DOI: 10.1007/978-3-642-59295-9

Springer-Verlag is a part of Springer Science+Business Media
springeronline.com
Product liability: The publisher cannot guarantee the accuracy of any information about dosage and application contained in this book. In every individual case the user must check such information by consulting the relevant literature.

Cover-Design: typographics GmbH, Darmstadt
Typesetting: typographics GmbH, Darmstadt

Printed on acid-free paper SPIN: 109 77 743 18/5141 5 4 3 2 1 0

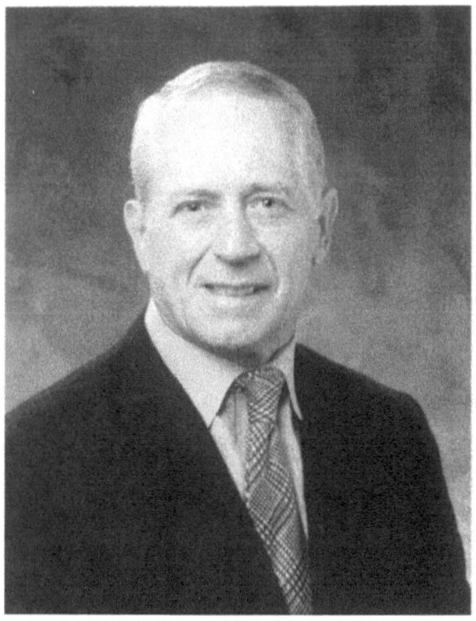

Leo A. Whiteside, M.D.
Missouri Bone and Joint Center
Biomechanical Research Laboratory
14825 Sugarwood Trail
St. Louis, MO 63014
USA

About the Author

Dr. Leo Whiteside, an internationally known orthopaedic surgeon-inventor and educator from St. Louis, Missouri, is recognized as one of the world's foremost authorities on osteointegration technology in total knee and hip arthroplasty. In the early 1980s he pioneered one of the first successful cementless total knee systems along with the first intramedullary alignment instrumentation system for knee surgery. He has designed three total hip systems, two total knee systems, and a unicondylar knee system. In the past decade he has dedicated much of his research effort to ligament balancing techniques in knee arthroplasty. After collecting and comparing extensive cadaveric laboratory and surgical-clinical data, he has developed protocols for balancing ligaments in primary and revision knees. As director of the Missouri Bone and Joint Center and its affiliated research foundation, Dr. Whiteside has published approximately 200 peer-reviewed journal articles and book chapters. He also serves on numerous orthopaedic committees and journal review boards.

Preface

Ligament balancing is an integral part of total knee arthroplasty, and remains thought - provoking and controversial years after alignment instrumentation and implants have been standardized. Although tensioning instruments have been used to guide the surgeon in bone surface resection, the compromises in alignment created by these instruments can lead to confounding problems with wear and patellar tracking.

The basic premise behind this book is that the knee must be both correctly aligned and balanced throughout the arc of flexion. In order to achieve these results the procedures must be accurate but also simple and quick to perform.

The general principle of alignment and ligament function should be understood thoroughly before the surgeon enters the operating room. This book was designed to impart a complete picture of how the alignment landmarks and ligament parameters work together, and to provide methods to address the abnormalities that occur as a result of deformity and ligament contracture. To receive the most benefit from this book the surgeon should first read the entire book to achieve a thorough understanding of the principles of alignment and ligament balancing. However, each chapter can be read and understood separately as a guide to pre-operation planning and as a technique manual in the operating room.

This book began as a surgical technique manual for use by fellows at the Missouri Bone and Joint Center in pre-operative planning and as a guide in the operating room. Because of demand for a manual for the orthopaedic surgeon who specializes in arthroplasty, a soft-cover edition was produced in English, and Springer-Verlag published a successful hard-bound edition in Italian. Now also a German Edition will be printed.

I would like to thank Scott Hartsell of Smith & Nephew for helping to start the process represented by this book, and for his continued support for surgical education, also to Andreas Hesse who helped to realize the German Edition. Also thanks should go to Springer-Verlag-Heidelberg, especially Thomas Guenther, for continuing to develop this surgical academic endeavor.

Leo A. Whiteside
Missouri Bone and Joint Center – Biomechanical Research Laboratory
St. Louis in January 2004

Table of Contents

1. Introduction

Although the knee has been studied intensively for decades, it continues to confound investigators and to frustrate surgeons. Its intricate ligaments and complex joint surfaces interact in ways that defy description. Nevertheless, the surgeon must repair and reconstruct the damaged and arthritic knee so that its performance is near normal, and this requires decisions and adjustments made with reasonable accuracy under the pressure and time constraints of the operating room. This book simplifies the geometry and kinematics of the knee enough that the knee can be understood and managed effectively. It establishes rules for resection and alignment that position the joint surfaces so that the ligaments can be balanced through the normal flexion arc, it illustrates stability tests that can be performed with ease, and it teaches safe guidelines for ligament release so that the ligament balancing can be performed quickly and effectively without destabilizing the knee.

The lower extremity often is depicted in two dimensions with the hip, knee, and ankle lying in a straight line, the -epi-condylar axis perpendicular to this line, and the joint line sloped downward medially.

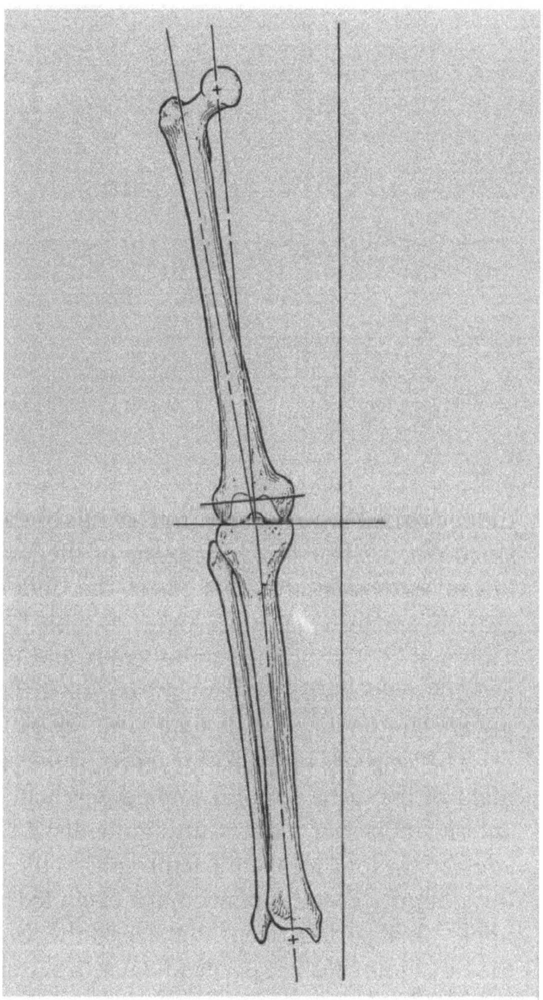

Fig. 1.
- The centers of the hip, knee, and ankle lie approximately in a straight line – the mechanical axis of the lower extremity.
- The mechanical axis of the femur is collinear with the mechanical axis of the lower extremity.
- The long axis of the femur (the anatomic axis) aligns in approx-imately 5° valgus to the mechanical axis of the lower extremity.
- The long axis of the tibia is collinear with the mechanical axis of the lower extremity.
- The patellar groove is collinear with the mechanical axis of the extremity and perpendicular to the epicondylar axis.

When depicted in three dimensions, the lower extremity functions in a plane throughout the flexion-extension arc, and the femoral head, the mechanical axis of the femur, the patellar groove, the inter-condylar notch, the patellar articular crest, the tibia, and the ankle remain within this plane. The axis through which the tibia rotates as the knee flexes and extends is perpendicular to this Median Anterior-Posterior Plane, and is approximated by the trans-epicondylar line, or epicondylar axis. The patella is drawn through the patellar groove, which also lies in the anterior-posterior plane.

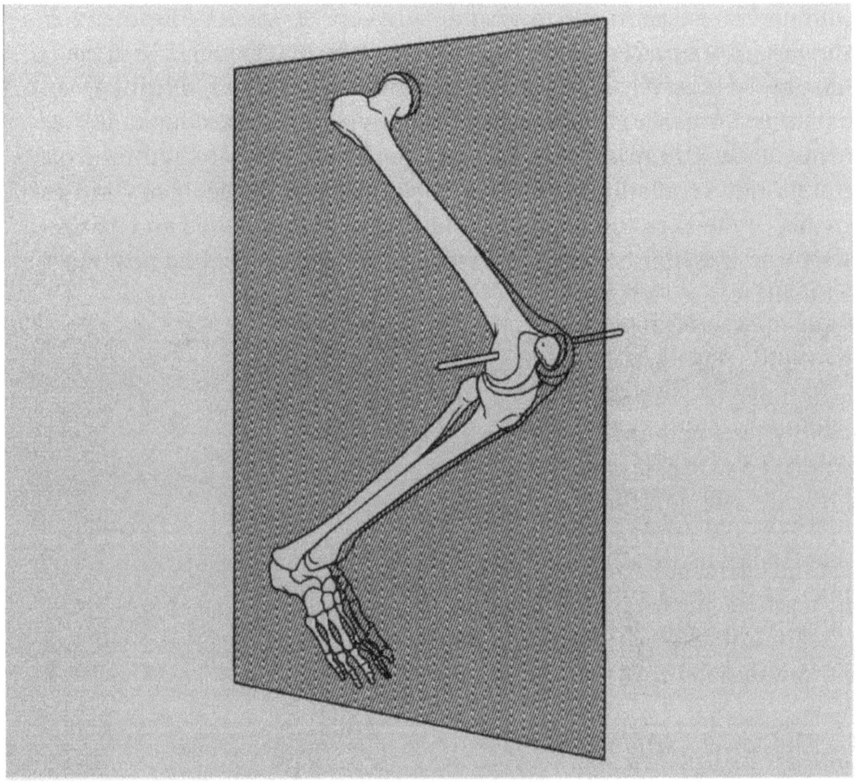

Fig. 2. The mechanical axis of the lower extremity becomes a plane when flexion and extension in three dimensions are considered. The centers of the hip, knee, and ankle remain within this plane through the flexion–extension arc. The patellar groove (anterior-posterior axis of the femur) is co-planar with this plane so that the patella is drawn smoothly through the groove as a rope is pulled smoothly through a well-aligned pulley. The epicondylar axis is perpendicular to the anterior-posterior plane, and the tibia swings through this axis, staying in the anterior-posterior plane throughout the flexion–extension arc.

In the normal knee the epicondylar axis of the femur remains perpendicular to the anterior-posterior plane of the lower extremity throughout the flexion-extension arc. This places the tibia nearly perpen-dicular to the ground, and also places the hip in its most favorable position for function. The joint surfaces between the femur and tibia are sloped downward toward the medial side on all weightbearing surfaces, which places them slightly in varus to the functional plane in all positions of flexion.

The long axis of the femur serves as the anatomical reference for alignment of the distal femoral cuts perpendicular to the mechanical axis and anterior-posterior plane. Cutting the distal femoral surfaces at a 5° valgus angle to the long axis of the femur places the joint surface perpendicular to the anterior-posterior plane in the extended position. Likewise, cutting the upper tibial surface perpendicular to the long axis of the tibia also places the tibial joint surface perpendicular to the anterior-posterior plane in extension.

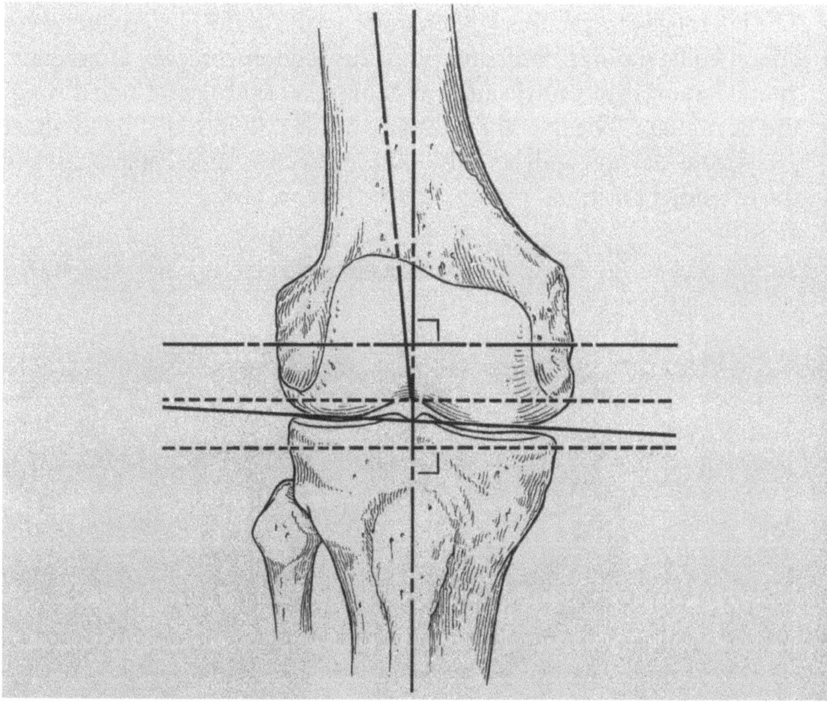

Fig. 3. In the extended position the joint surface slopes medially approximately 3°.
– Tibial resection is perpendicular to the long axis of the tibia and mechanical axis of the lower extremity. The resection surface is 3° valgus to the articular surface.
– Femoral resection is perpendicular to the mechanical axis, and 5° valgus to the long axis of the femur. The resection surface is approximately 3° varus to the articular surface.
– These 3° "errors" in the femoral and tibial surface resections compensate for one another, and result in surface resections that are parallel to one another and perpendicular to the mechanical axis of the lower extremity.

The anterior-posterior axis serves as the anatomic landmark for femoral resection in flexion. The anterior-posterior axis can be constructed by marking the lateral edge of the posterior cruciate ligament and the deepest part of the patellar groove. A line drawn between these two points lies in the anterior-posterior plane and passes through the center of the femoral head and down the long axis of the tibia.

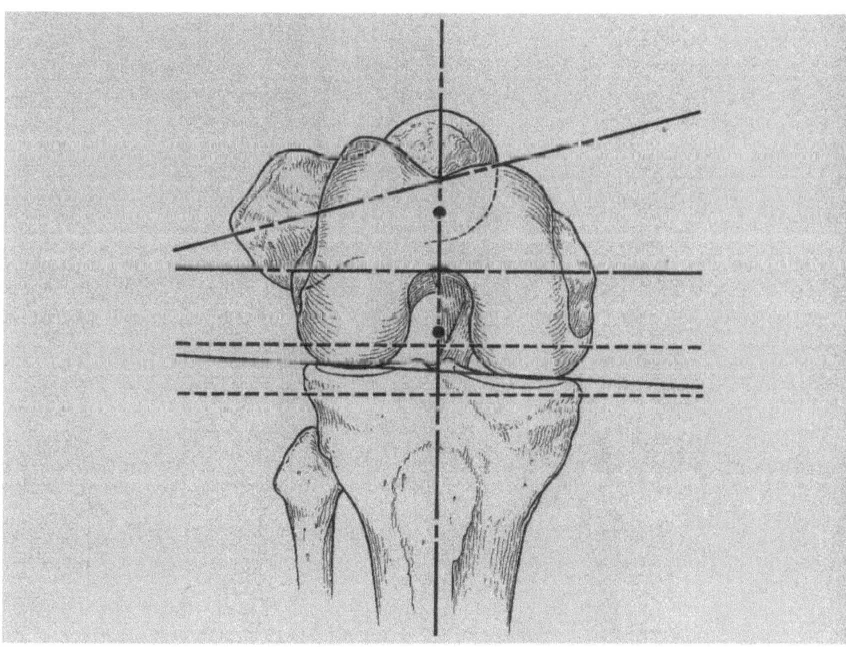

Fig. 4. With the knee flexed 90°, the joint surface resections are parallel to the epi condylar axis and perpendicular to the anterior-posterior axis of the femur. The femoral neck is anteverted approximately 15° to the epicondy-lar axis. When the knee is in functional position in flexion (walking up stairs or standing from a seated position), the positions of the femoral neck and epicondylar axis remain unchanged, and in the normal knee the tibia is vertical.

The lateral gastrocnemius tendon and capsule of the posterolateral corner, lateral collateral ligament, and popliteus tendon complex attach near the lateral femoral epicondyle and are stabilizers of the lateral side throughout the flexion arc. The lateral posterior capsule and iliotibial band attach far away from the epicondylar axis and are effective lateral stabilizers only in the extended position.

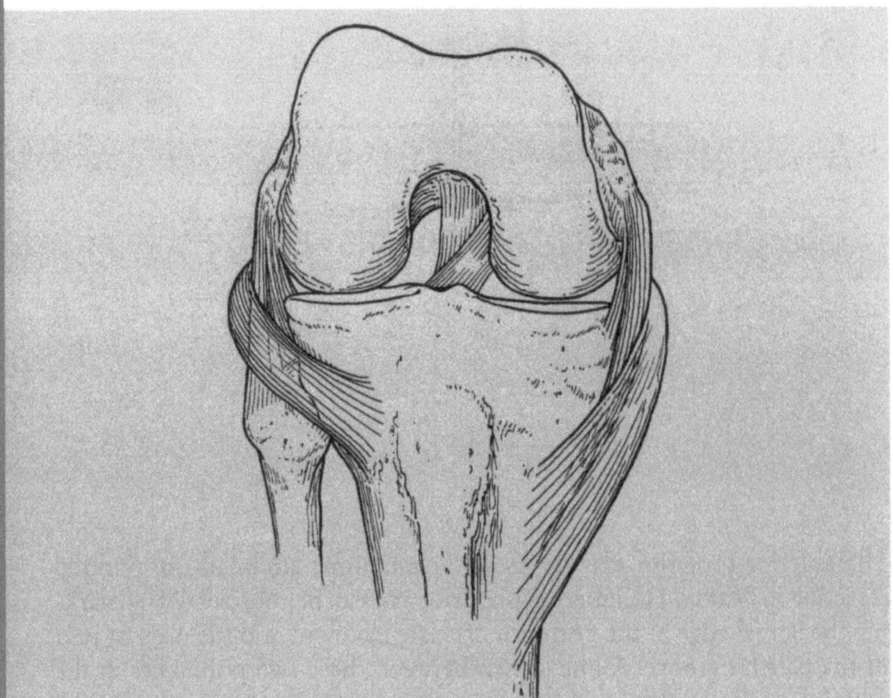

Fig. 5. With the knee flexed and viewed from anteriorly, the deep and superficial medial collateral ligament fibers stabilize the medial side. The lateral collateral ligament and popliteus tendon stabilize the lateral side, and the posterior cruciate ligament is a secondary varus and valgus stabilizing structure. The pes anserinus and iliotibial band are parallel to the joint and do not afford medial or lateral stability in the flexed position.

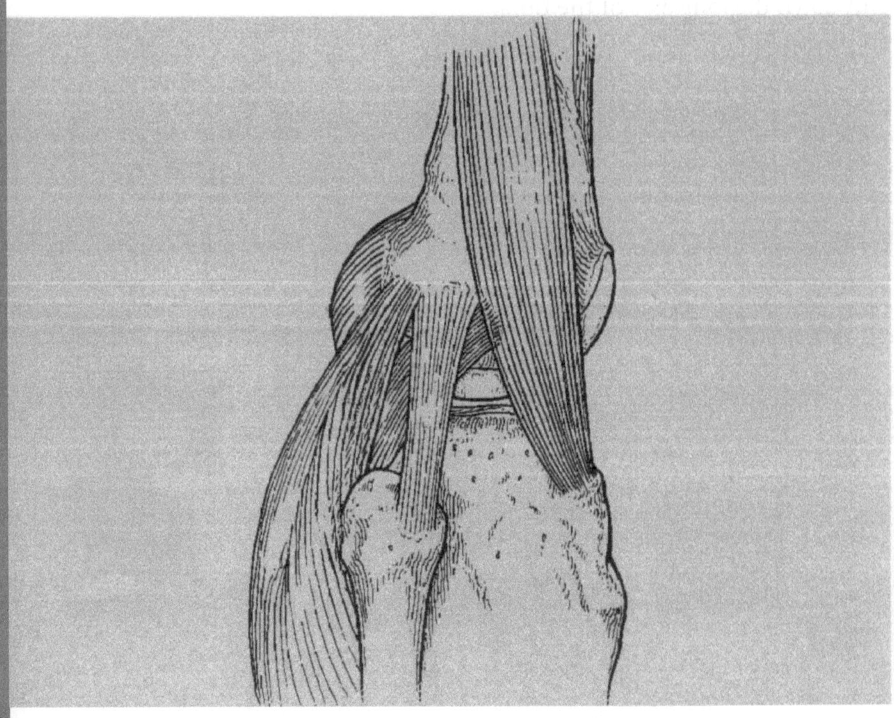

Fig. 6. Lateral view of the knee showing the major lateral static stabilizing structures with the knee extended. The lateral gastrocnemius tendon (and posterolateral corner capsule), lateral collateral ligament, lateral posterior capsule, popliteus tendon, and iliotibial band all cross the joint perpendicular (or nearly so) to its surface, and are capable of stabilizing the knee in the extended position.

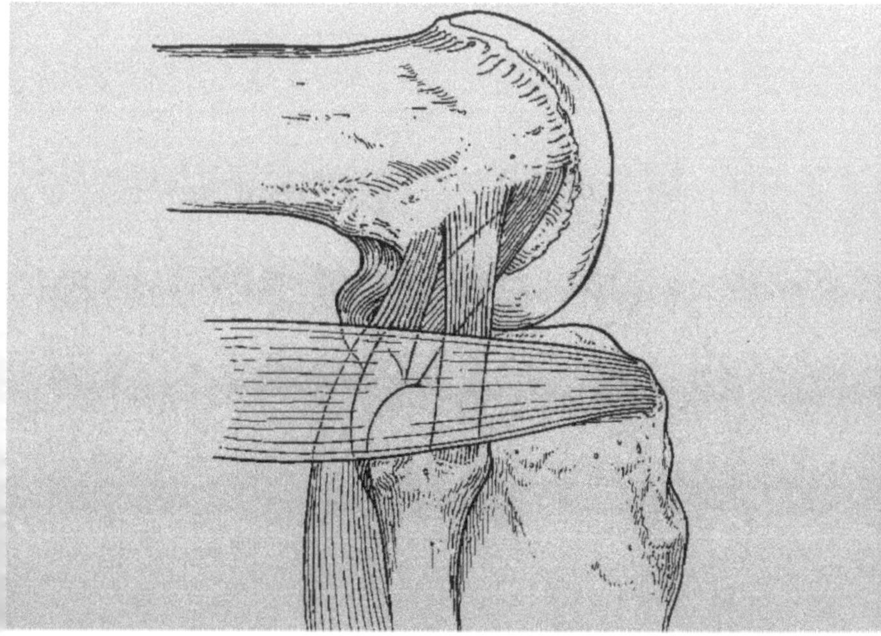

Fig. 7. Lateral view of the knee showing the major lateral static stabilizing structures with the knee flexed 90°. The lateral gastrocnemius tendon, posterolateral corner capsule, lateral collateral ligament, and popliteus tendon are the only effective lateral stabilizing structures with the knee flexed to this position. The iliotibial band is parallel to the joint surface, and the lateral posterior capsule is slack.

On the medial side, the medial collateral ligament (anterior and posterior portions) is attached to the epicondyle, and is effective throughout the flexion arc. The epicondylar attachment is broad enough that there is a difference in function of the anterior and posterior portions of this ligament in flexion and extension. The medial posterior capsule attaches far from the epicondylar axis, and is tight only in extension. The posterior cruciate ligament is attached slightly distal and posterior to the epicondylar axis, so it slackens in full extension and tightens in flexion.

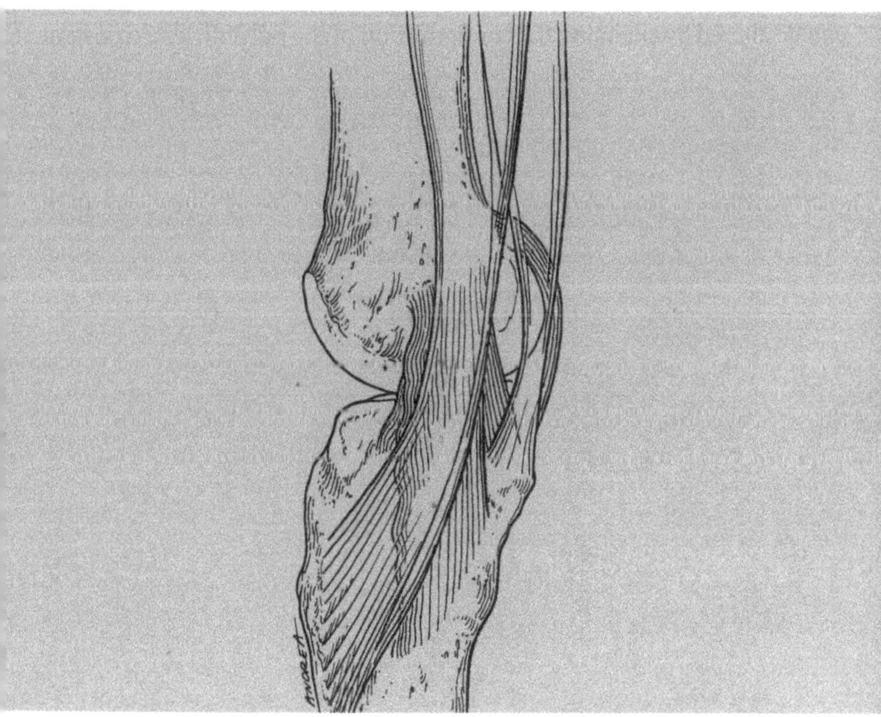

Fig. 8. On the medial view, the medial collateral ligament (deep and superficial) is the primary medial stabilizer that is tight in extension. The anterior fibers are slackened in full extension and the posterior fibers (posteromedial oblique ligament) are differentially tightened in extension because of their position in the medial femoral condyle. The lateral posterior-capsule also is tight. Active medial stability is added by the medial hamstrings through the pes anserinus and semimembranosus.

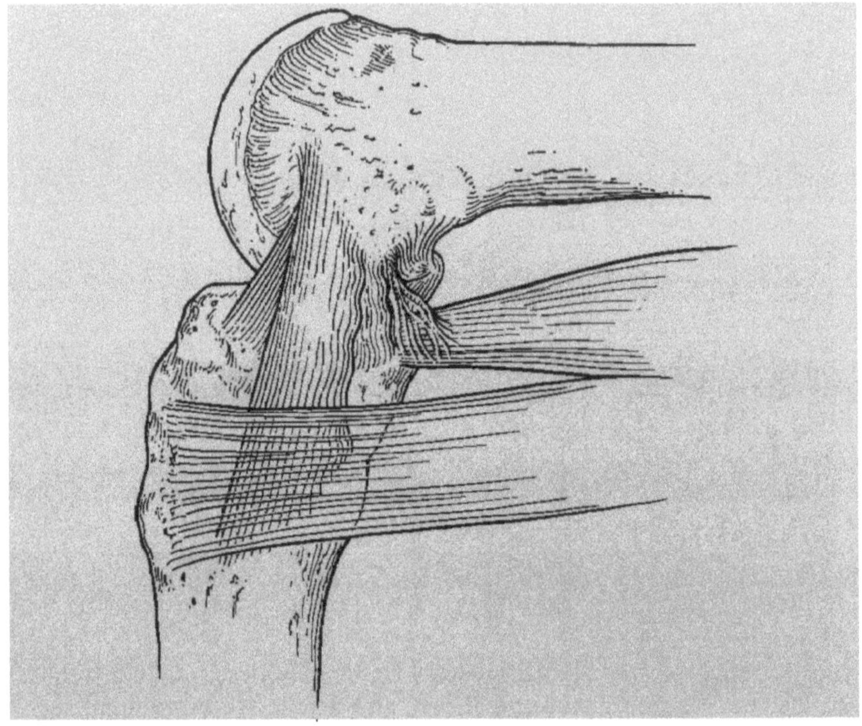

Fig. 9. Viewed from the medial side with the knee flexed, the medial stabilizing structures are the deep and superficial medial collateral ligament. The anterior fibers of the medial collateral ligament are taut and the posterior fibers are relatively lax because of their attach-ment more posteriorly on the femur. The posterior capsule is slack and is not effective in flexion. The semi-membranosus and pes anserina are parallel with the joint and are incapable of supplying active stability in flexion.

Knowing this information, the surgeon can, after positioning the implants properly with the axes of the knee, assess knee stability in flexion and extension and release the structures that are tight. The surgeon also can adjust the tightness of intact ligaments by changing the position and size of the femoral component, altering the slope of the tibial surfaces, and adjusting the thickness of the tibial polyethylene spacers. Anterior-posterior stability can be altered by changing the configuration of the polyethylene component.

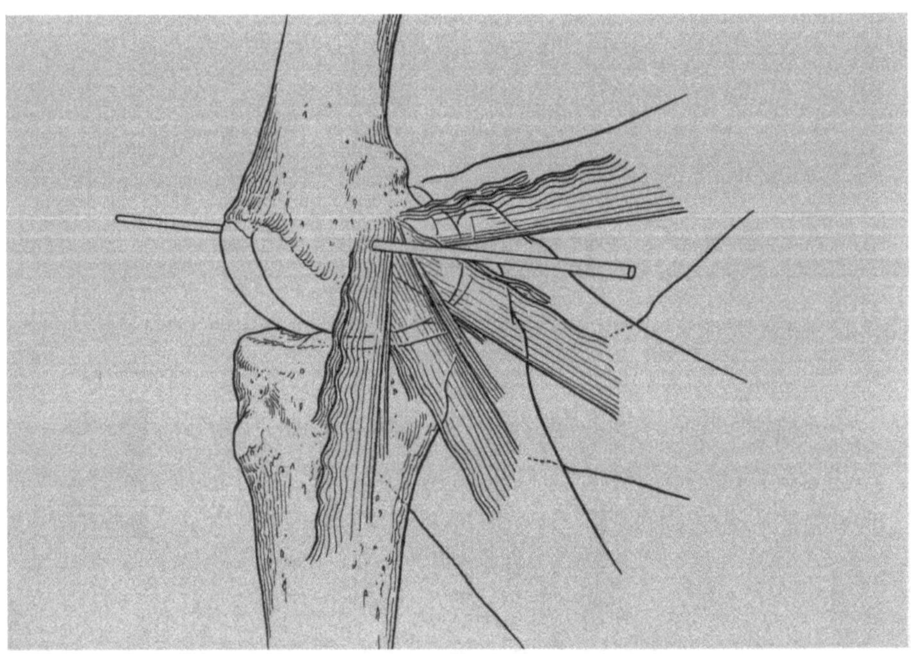

Fig. 10. Ligaments that attach to the femur near the epicondyles guide the tibia through its arc of flexion and maintain stability throughout the full range of motion. Because the ligaments attach across a finite surface of the condyles, the anterior and posterior portions behave differently in flexion and extension. As illustrated in this drawing, the anterior portion of the medial collateral ligament tightens in flexion, and the posterior portion tightens in extension.

The arthritic process often affects the articular surfaces and ligaments to cause deformity, and this places the tibia outside the functional plane. To achieve optimal function of the knee in flexion and extension, the joint surfaces must be returned to their proper positions and the liga-ments adjusted to their proper tensions through-out the functional arc of the knee.

A number of factors in the arthritic process affect the functions of ligaments. Osteophytes deform them, causing them to be excessively tight, or restrict sliding, causing flexion contracture and restriction of flexion. As the joint surfaces collapse, their attachment points come closer together and the ligaments shorten irreversibly. When the joint surfaces separate on the convex side of a deformity, the ligaments usually are elongated permanently. All these abnormalities can be addressed by thorough debridement of the joint, choice of size and position of the implants, and release of contracted ligaments.

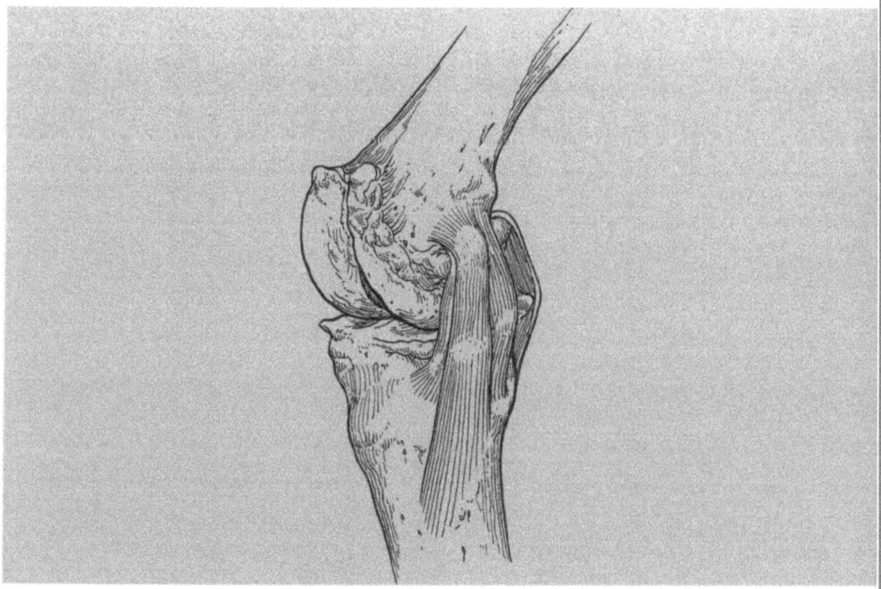

Fig. 11. Osteophytes are an important factor in ligament balancing. They constrain the deep and superficial medial collateral ligament and the medial posterior capsule.

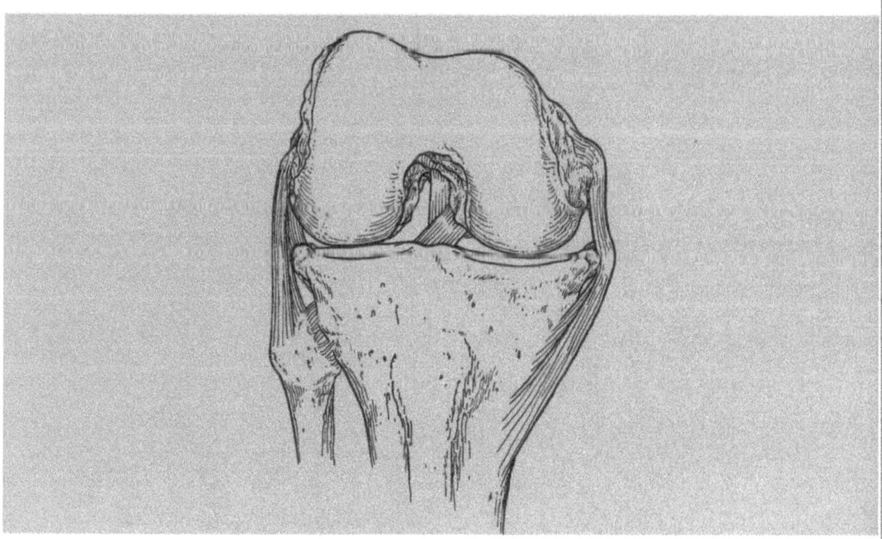

Fig. 12. Osteophytes surround the posterior cruciate ligament and interfere with flexion and extension, and also invade the popliteus recess, restricting flexibility on the lateral side of the knee.

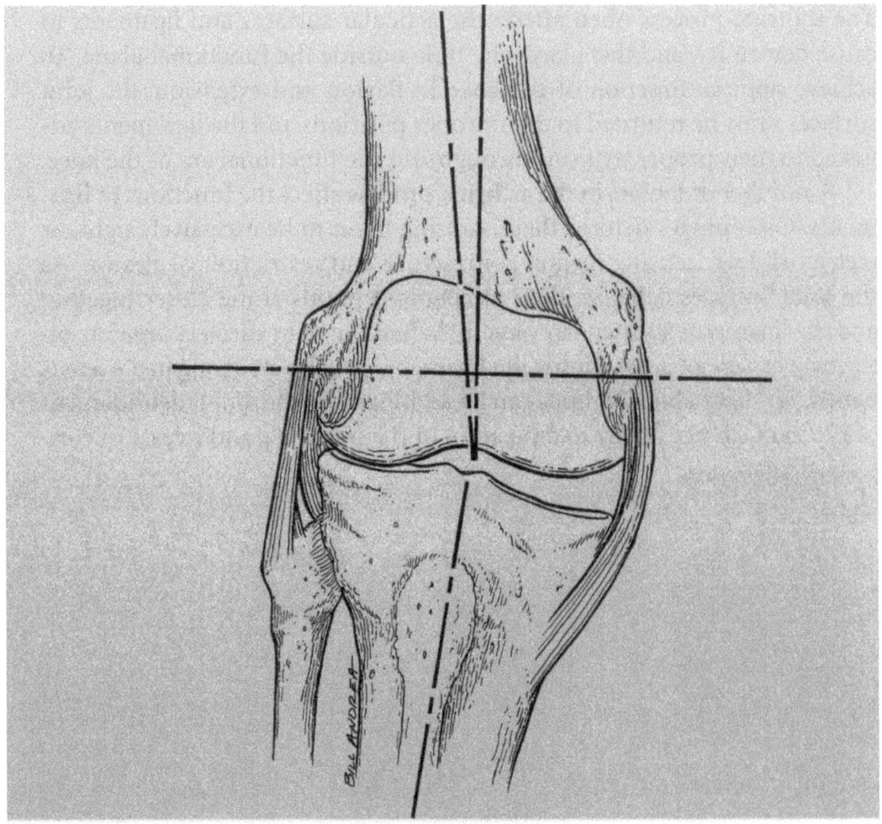

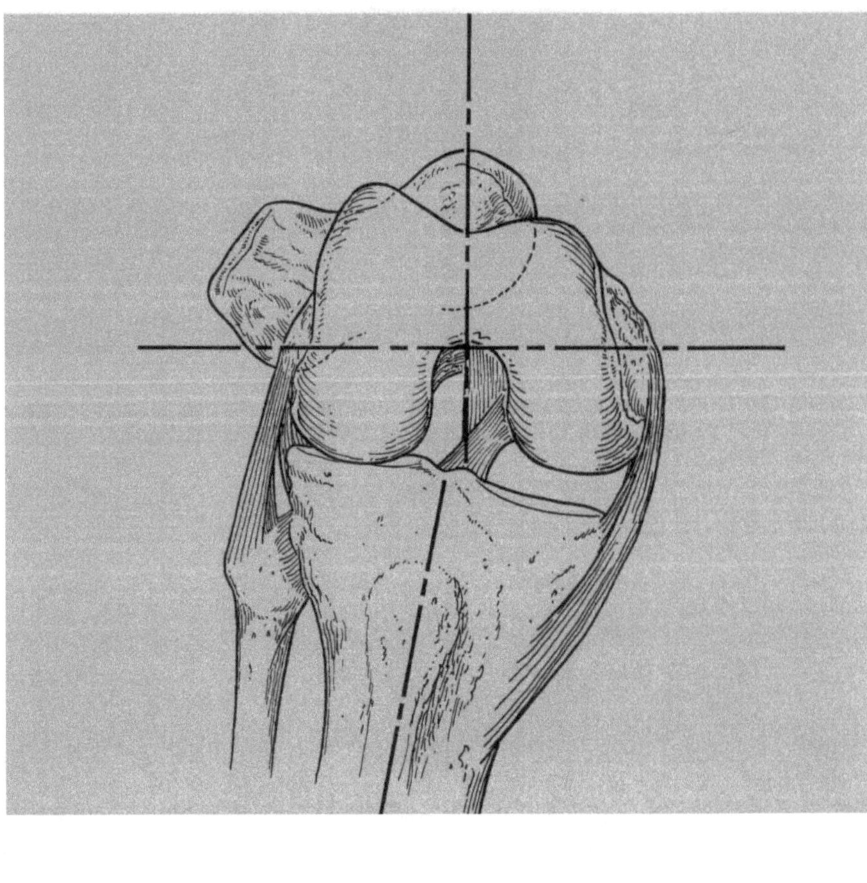

Fig. 13, 14. When all medial and lateral stabilizers that are attached to the epicondyles are deformed (either stretched or contracted) the deformity is effective throughout the flexion–extension arc. In these illustrations the lateral collateral ligament and popliteus tendon are contracted, causing the knee to be tight laterally both in flexion and extension. The anterior and posterior portions of the medial collateral ligament are stretched so the knee is loose medially in flexion and extension.

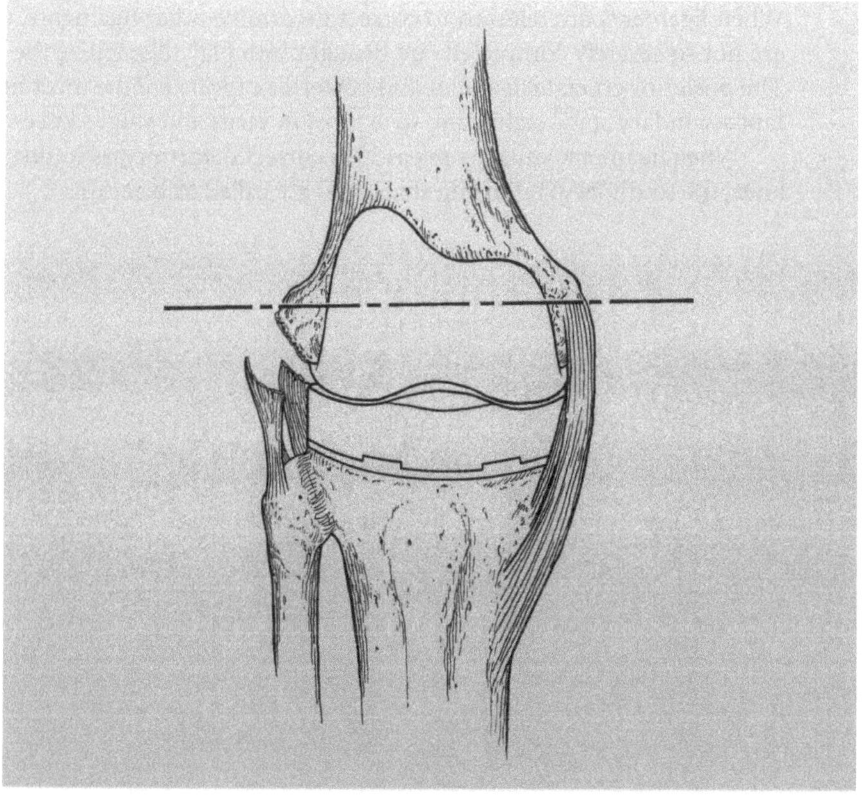

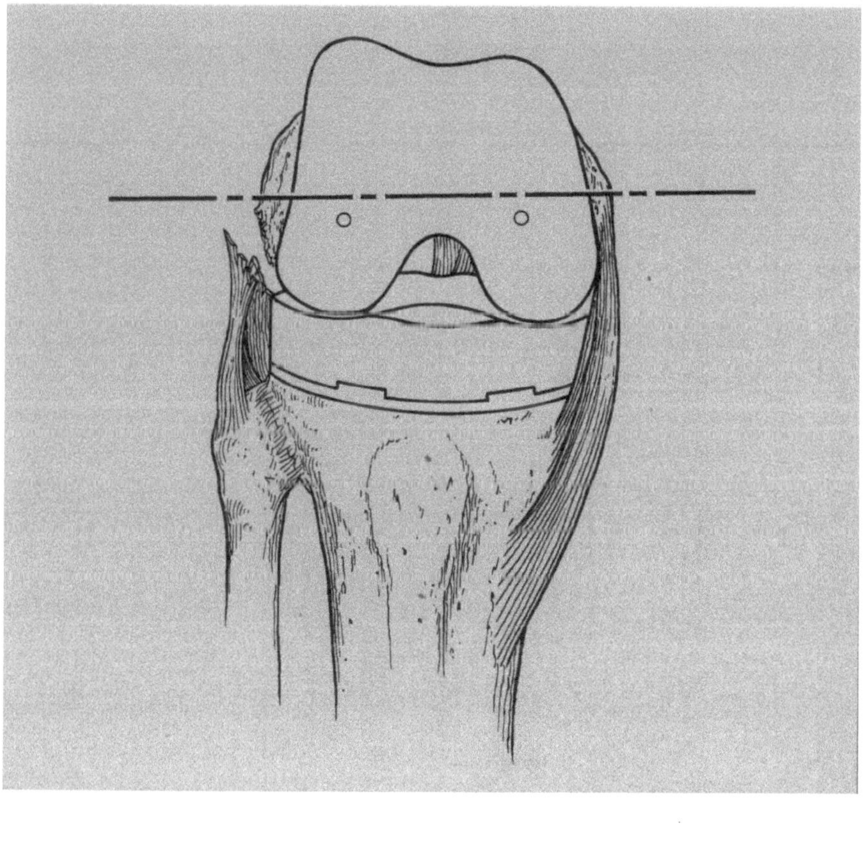

Fig. 15, 16. Release of the lateral collateral ligament and popliteus tendon has a similar effect in flexion and extension. Likewise, addition of thickness to the tibia restores medial stability similarly in flexion and extension.

When ligaments are released to correct deformity, other ligaments, which are not so severely contracted, are brought into play to stabilize the knee. The posterior cruciate ligament and posterior capsule are the most important secondary static stabilizing structures in varus and valgus knees.

When ligaments must be released to correct deformity, as in this varus knee, the secondary stabilizing structures are called into action.

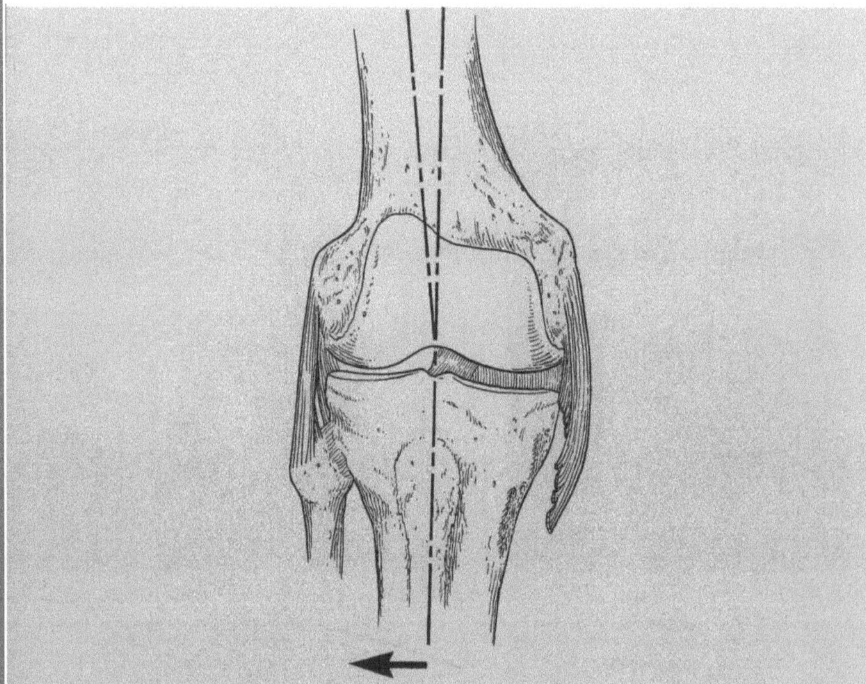

Fig. 17. Release of the anterior and posterior portions of the medial collateral ligament leaves the knee dependent on the medial posterior capsule for medial stability in extension.

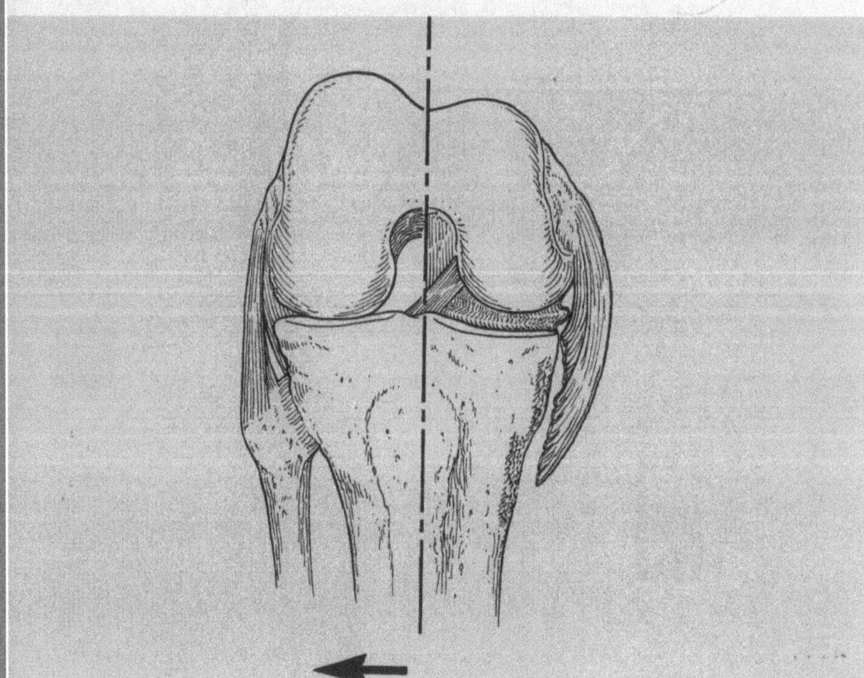

Fig. 18. In flexion, the medial posterior capsule is lax, so the knee is especially dependent on the posterior cruciate ligament for medial stability in flexion after release of the medial collateral ligament.

Contracture or elongation of these secondary stabilizing structures may affect ligament balance as well, and sometimes these structures must be adjusted. Because the posterior cruciate ligament is a medial structure, it often is contracted in the varus knee and stretched in the valgus knee.

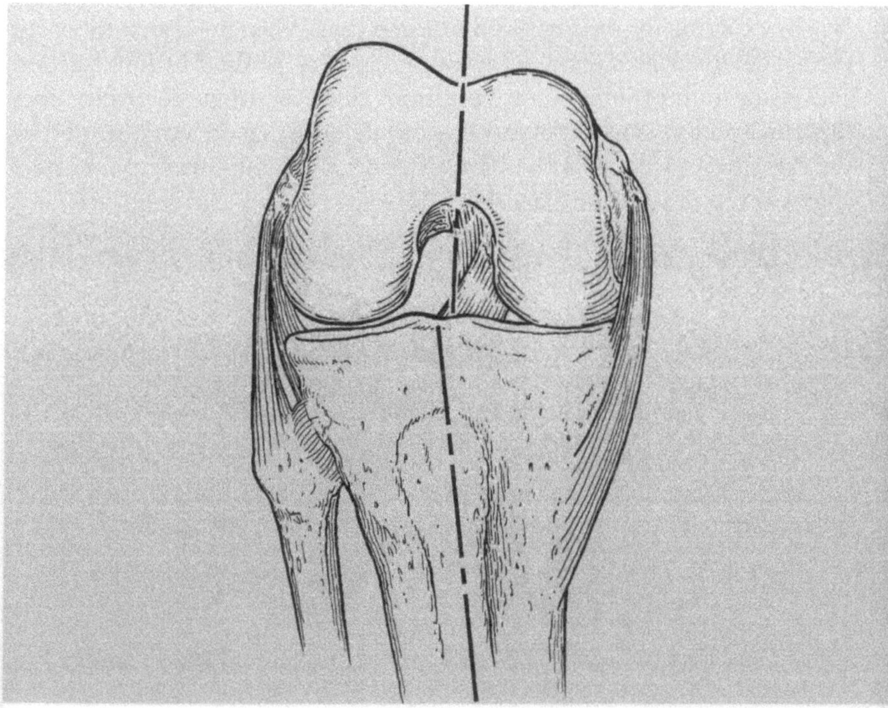

Fig. 19. The posterior cruciate ligament is a medial structure, and often is contracted in the varus knee along with the medial collateral ligament. Thus it often must be released in the varus knee.

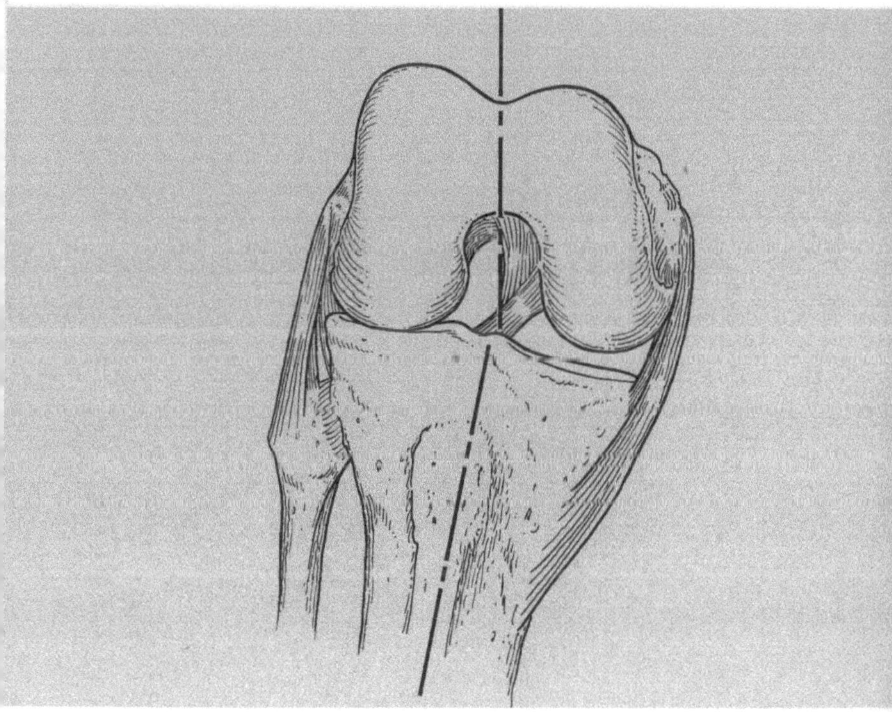

Fig. 20. The medial position of the posterior cruciate ligament makes it vulnerable to stretching in the valgus knee. Thus it often must be substituted for in the valgus knee.

In the knee that is free of deformity in which there is no ligament contracture or stretching of ligaments, resection of the thickness of the implant from all surfaces and replacement of this thickness of bone with the implant results in restoration of ligament balance through the full flexion arc. This statement is intuitively obvious and also has been demonstrated to be true by experiment (see suggested readings list). When no deformity exists, the articular surfaces them-selves can be used as landmarks for resection and restoration of joint surface position. However, when deformity does exist, anatomical landmarks and axes of reference that are not distorted by the arthritic process must be used to resect the bone surfaces in correct alignment in flexion and extension.

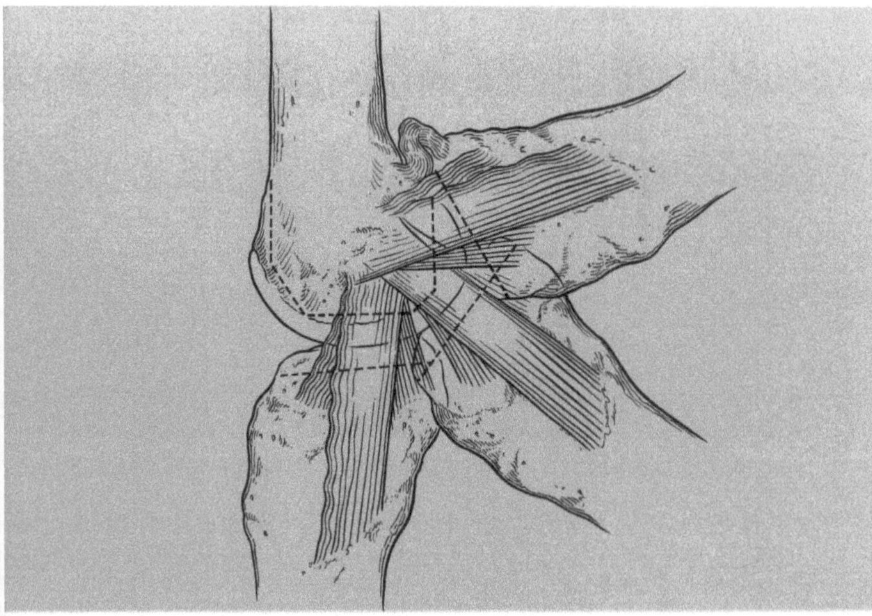

Fig. 21. As the tibial articular surface slides on the curved surface of the femur, the ligaments that attach to the epicondyles maintain normal tension through the flexion arc due to the shape of the femoral condyles and tibial surface. Resection of the thickness of the implants from the distal and posterior surfaces of the femur and from the upper surface of the tibia prepares the knee for replacement so that the ligaments will function correctly through the full arc of flexion.

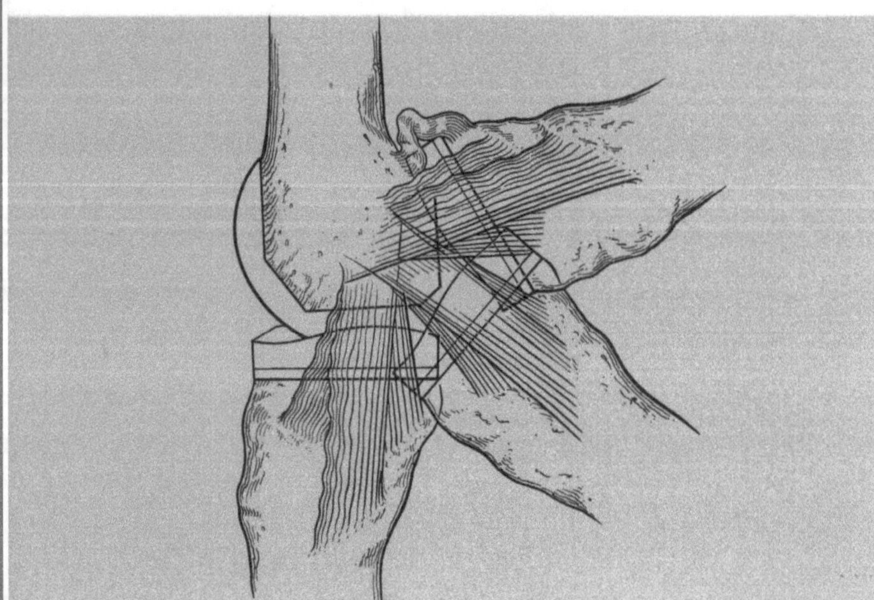

Fig. 22. Replacement of these resected surfaces with the total knee replacement components leaves the ligaments performing normally through the full flexion arc.

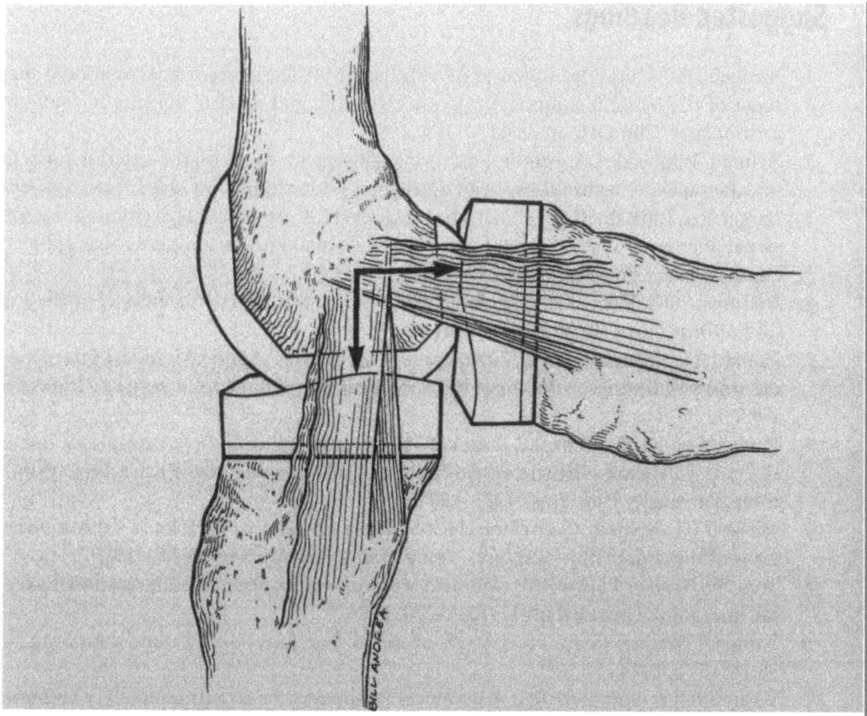

Fig. 23. In most cases the intact (convex) side of the knee should serve as the landmark for resection both distally and posteriorly. Even when the collateral ligaments are stretched, the distal and posterior surfaces will be positioned correctly to accept a thicker tibial component to achieve stability in flexion and extension, and the ligaments on the contracted (concave) side can be released to achieve correct balance to accommodate this position.

Restoration of the joint surfaces to their proper alignment with the mechanical axes of the extremity is the cornerstone of successful ligament balance, stability, and kinematics of the knee in total knee arthroplasty. This is accomplished by aligning the joint surfaces perpendicular to the anterior-posterior plane, and the simplest means of establishing the position of the anterior-posterior plane is to establish the mechanical axis of the lower extremity in flexion and extension. The mechanical axis of the femur in extension is estimated easily by placing a rod down the femoral shaft. Then the bone is resected at a 5° valgus angle to this rod. The mechanical axis of the femur in flexion is estimated easily by a line drawn in the anterior-posterior axis of the femur, and the bone is resected perpendicular to this line. The tibial shaft lies in the anterior-posterior plane in flexion and extension, so the tibial joint surface is resected perpendicular to the long axis of the tibia. This can be established with either an intramedullary rod or an extramedullary guide. By using the three accessible anatomic axes, the femoral and tibial components can be positioned so that the knee is in correct varus-valgus alignment throughout the flexion arc. The ligaments then can be balanced around the joint by determining which ligaments are contracted based on their function in flexion and extension. Simply stated, ligaments that attach to the femur on or near the epicondyles are effective both in flexion and extension, and those that attach distant from the epicondylar axis are effective either in flexion or extension, but not in both positions. To extend this concept further, it can be stated that the portions of the ligament complexes that attach anteriorly in the epi-condylar areas stabilize primarily in flexion, and those that attach posteriorly in the epicondylar areas stabilize primarily in extension.

Suggested Readings

1. Anouchi YS, Whiteside LA, Kaiser AD, Milliano MT: The effect of axial rotational alignment of the femoral component on knee stability and patellar tracking in total knee arthroplasty. Clin Orthop 287:170–177, 1991.
2. Arima J, Whiteside LA: Femoral rotational alignment, based on the anterior-posterior axis, in total knee arthroplasty in a valgus knee. J Bone Joint Surg 77A:1331–1334, 1995.
3. Berger RA, Rubash HE, Seel MJ, Thompson WH, Crossett LS: Determining the rotational alignment of the femoral component in total knee arthroplasty using the epicondylar axis. Clin Orthop 286:40–49, 1993.
4. Brantigan OC, Voshell AF: The mechanics of the ligaments and menisci of the knee joint. J Bone Joint Surg 23:44–66, 1941.
5. Cooke TD, Pichora D, Siu D, Scudamore RA, Bryant JT: Surgical implications of varus deformity of the knee with obliquity of joint surfaces. J Bone Joint Surg Br 71:560–565, 1989.
6. Hungerford DS, Krackow KA, Kenna RV: Alignment in total knee arthroplasty. In Dorr LD (ed). The Knee – Papers of the First Scientific Meeting of the Knee Society. Baltimore, University Park Press 9–21, 1985.
7. Markolf KL, Mensch JS, Amstutz HC: Stiffness and laxity of the knee – the contributions of the supporting structures. J Bone Joint Surg Am 58:583–594, 1976.
8. Trent PS, Walker PS, Wolf B: Ligament length patterns, strength and rotational axes of the knee joint. Clin Orthop 117:263–270, 1976.
9. Wang CJ, Walker PS: Rotatory laxity of the human knee joint. J Bone Joint Surg Am: 56:161–170, 1974.
10. Whiteside LA, Summers RG: Anatomical landmarks for an intramedullary alignment system for total knee replacement. Orthop Trans 7:546–547, 1983.
11. Whiteside LA, Summers RG: The effect of the level of distal femoral resection on ligament balance in total knee replacement. In Dorr LD (ed). The Knee: Papers of the First Scientific Meeting of the Knee Society. Baltimore, University Park Press 59–73, 1984.
12. Whiteside LA, Kasselt MR, Haynes DW: Varus-valgus and rotational stability in rotationally unconstrained total knee arthroplasty. Clin Orthop 219:147–157, 1987.
13. Whiteside LA, McCarthy DS: Laboratory evaluation of alignment and kinematics in a unicompartmental knee arthroplasty inserted with intramedullary instrumentation. Clin Orthop 274:238–247, 1992.
14. Whiteside LA, Arima J: The anterior-posterior axis for femoral rotational alignment in valgus total knee arthroplasty. Clin Orthop 321:168–172, 1995.
15. Yoshii I, Whiteside LA, White SE, Milliano MT: Influence of prosthetic joint line position on knee kinematics and patellar position. J Arthroplasty 6:169–177, 1991.
16. Yoshioka Y, Siu D, Cooke TDV: The anatomy and functional axes of the femur. J Bone Joint Surg Am 69:873–880, 1987.
17. Yoshioka Y, Cooke TDV: Femoral anteversion: Assessment based on function axes. J Orthop Res 5:86–91, 1987.

Patella

2. Patella

Basic Principles

The patella maintains a delicate balance in total knee arthroplasty, and is dependent on position and configuration of the patellar and femoral articular surfaces, angle of the quadriceps and patellar tendons, and tension of the medial and lateral retinacula. As the knee flexes, the patella engages the patellar groove and then follows this groove through the flexion arc. The apex of the patella stays within the median anterior-posterior plane in the normal knee, and the patellar groove also must lie in this plane to accommodate this patellar position.

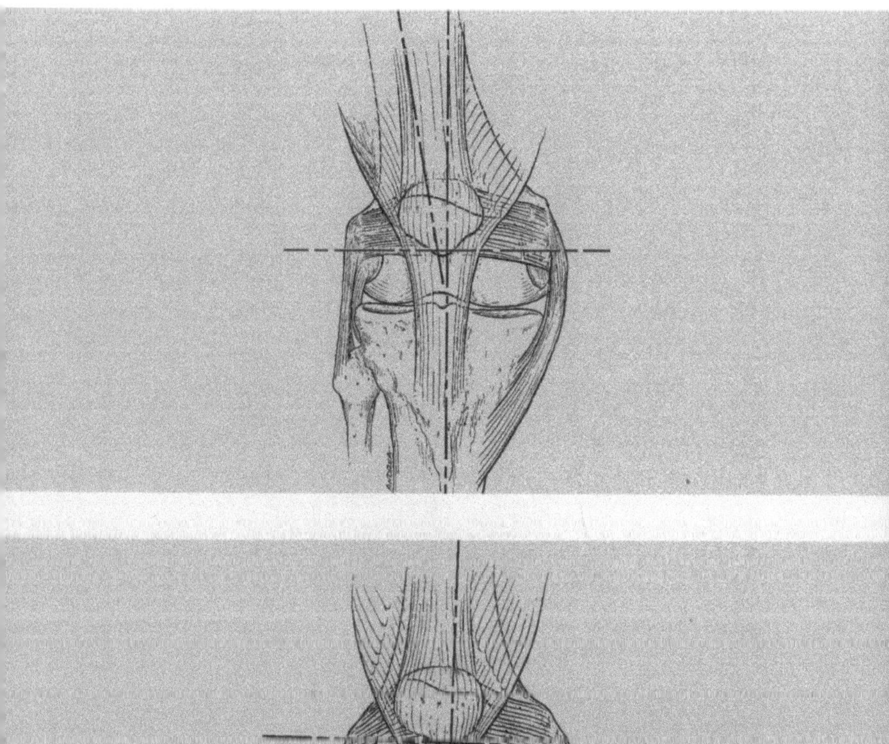

Fig. 24. In the normal knee the patellar crest lies about equidistant from the medial and lateral epicondyles. The lateral facet is wider than the medial facet, so the patella and patellar tendon lie slightly lateral to the midline. The medial and lateral retinacular structures are somewhat loose in extension.

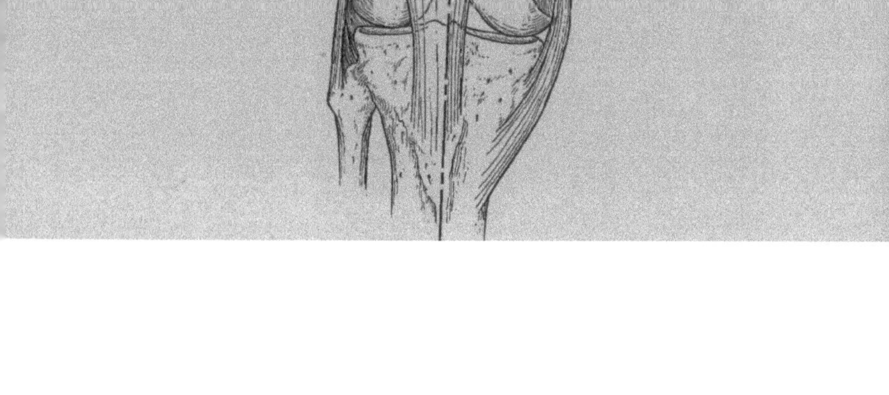

Fig. 25. As the knee flexes the patella stays in the patellar groove and thus follows the anterior-posterior plane of the femur. The medial and lateral retinacula begin to tighten as the knee flexes.

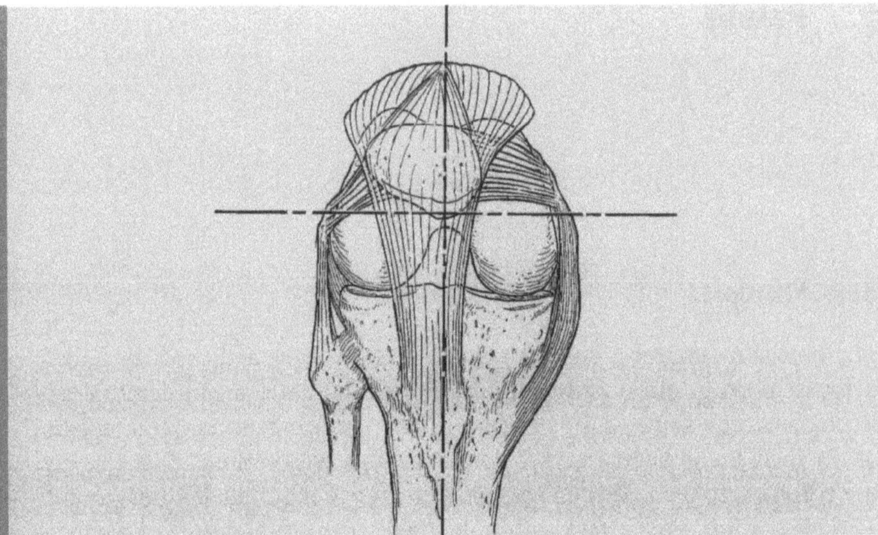

Fig. 26. As the knee continues to flex the patella is drawn along in the patellar groove as a rope is drawn through a pulley. The medial and lateral retinacula tighten even more.

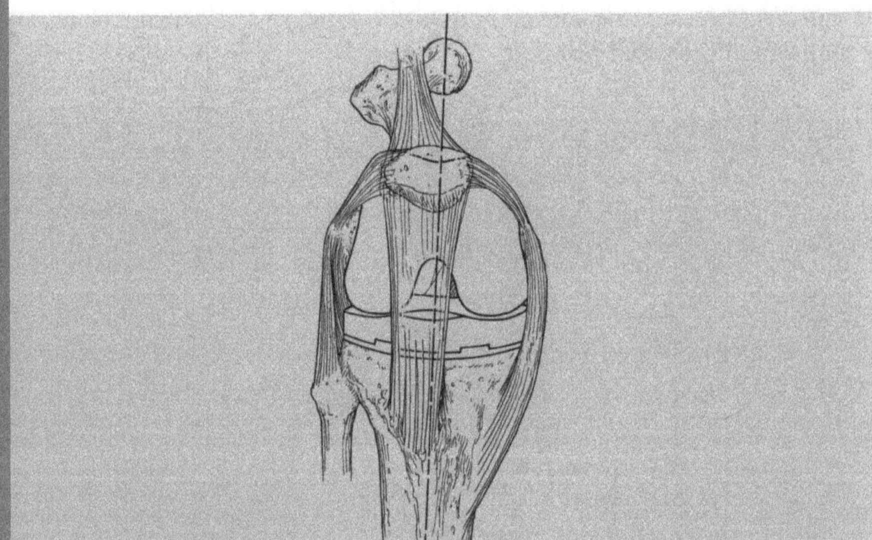

Fig. 27. Correct resection of the femoral surfaces is necessary to achieve stable patellar function through the entire arc of flexion. When the femoral component is aligned correctly with the anterior-posterior plane, the joint surfaces are perpendicular to the anterior-posterior axis in flexion. The patella is held in position by the contour of the patellar groove, which also is co-planar with the anterior-posterior plane, and by the tension in the quadriceps, patellar tendon, and medial and lateral patellar retinacula.

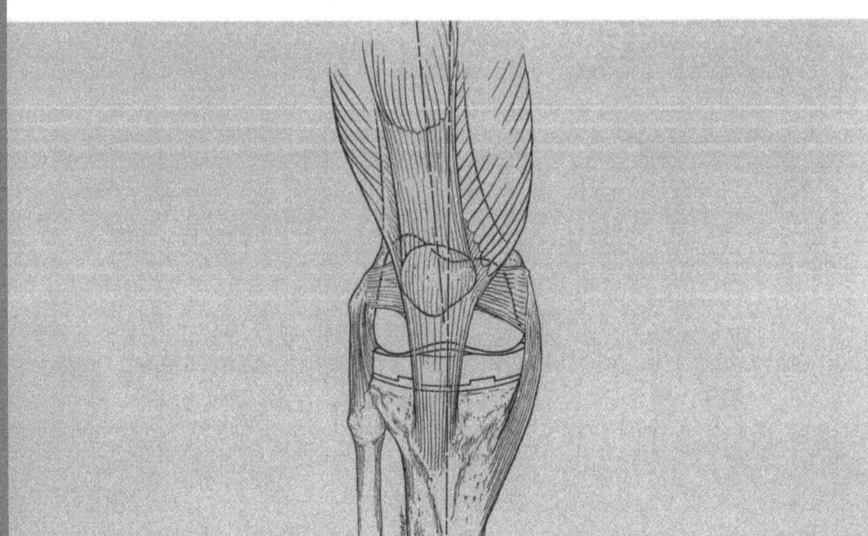

Fig. 28. In the extended position, the patellar groove is equidistant from the medial and lateral epicondyles and lies in the median anterior-posterior plane. The joint surfaces are perpendicular to the median anterior-posterior plane. The tibial tubercle is lateral to the midline anterior-posterior plane in all degrees of flexion, so the pressure is always greater on the lateral side of the patella, and there is a tendency for the patella to sublux laterally. Thus it is necessary to have a deep patellar groove and an elevated lateral flange surface.

Displacement of the patellar groove from its normal position and alignment in the midline anterior-posterior plane causes abnormalities in all the mechanisms that stabilize patellar tracking. Placing the femoral component in internal rotation relative to the median anterior-posterior plane malaligns the patellar groove with the line of pull of the quadriceps mechanism, and has the same effect as malaligning a pulley with the rope that is pulled through it. Therefore, when the femoral component is internally rotated, the quadriceps mechanism becomes unstable in the groove.

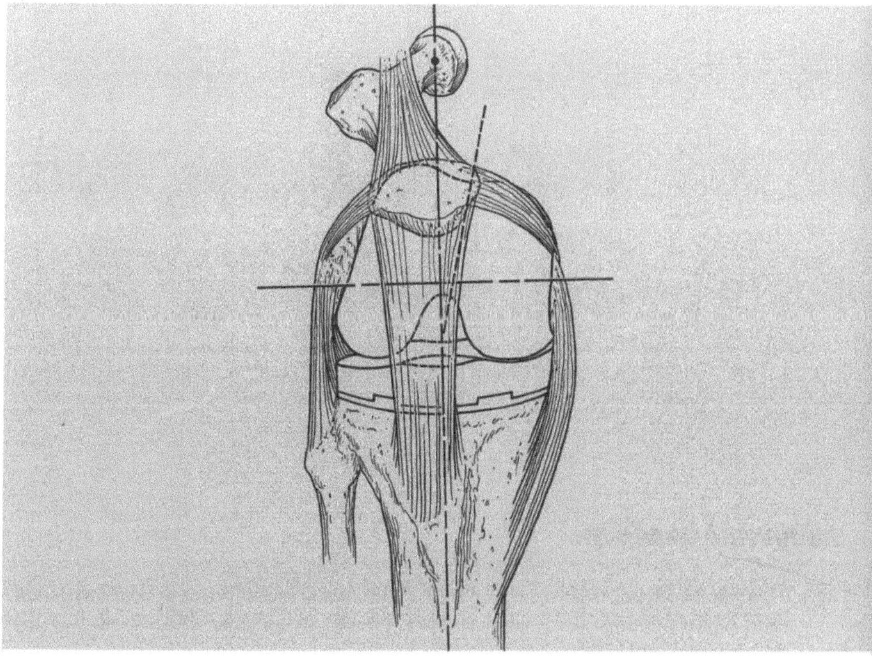

Fig. 29. Internal rotational malposition of the femoral component medializes the patellar groove and presents the patella with a slanted track in which to run. It also aligns the knee in valgus in flexed positions. As depicted here, the knee is not bearing load, so the lateral joint gapes open, and the tibia remains aligned with the anterior-posterior plane of the lower extremity.

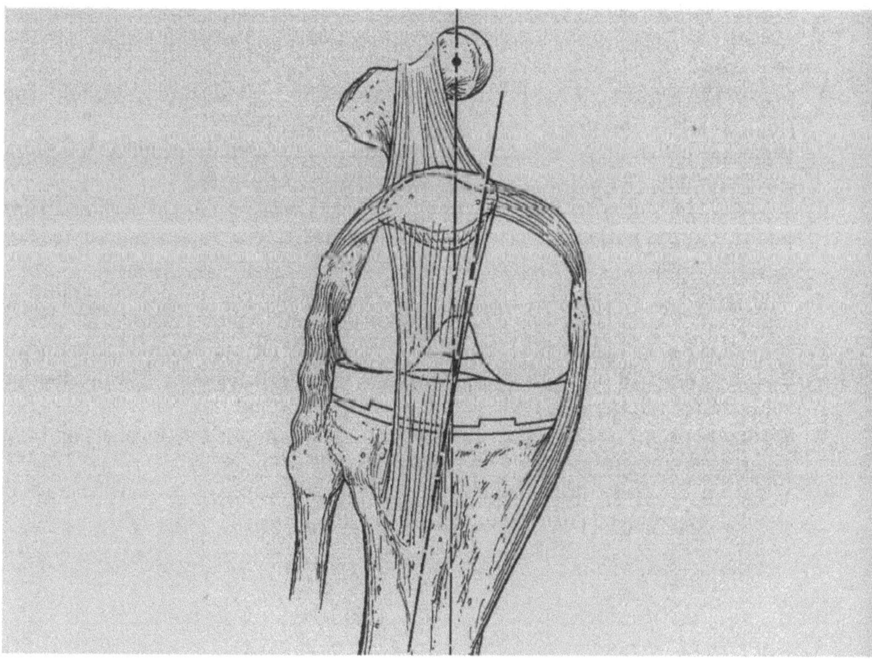

Fig. 30. When, on weight bearing, the tibia collapses into the valgus position dictated by the position of the femoral component, the tibial tubercle shifts laterally, increasing the Q-angle, thus increasing the lateralizing force on the patella, and worsening the tendency for the patella to sublux laterally. Now the tibia is aligned with the patellar groove, but neither the tibia nor the patellar groove is aligned with the anterior-posterior plane of the lower extremity.

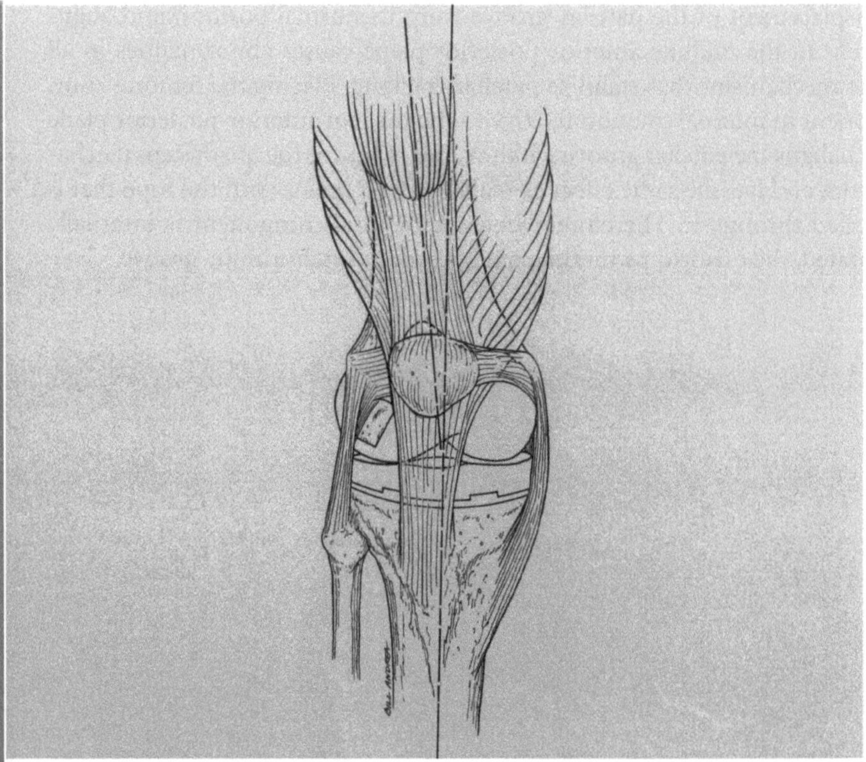

Fig. 31. With the knee in the extended position, the knee joint is in correct varus-valgus alignment, but the femoral component is internally rotated. This malposition of the femoral component medializes the patellar groove while leaving the epicondyles, patellar retinacula, and patella in their normal positions. Therefore the patella is subluxed laterally in extension.

Suggested Readings

1. Anouchi YS, Whiteside LA, Kaiser AD, Milliano MT: The effect of axial rotational alignment of the femoral component on knee stability and patellar tracking in total knee arthroplasty. Clin Orthop 287:170–177, 1991.
2. Arima J, Whiteside LA: Femoral rotational alignment, based on the anterior-posterior axis, in total knee arthroplasty in a valgus knee. J Bone Joint Surg 77A:1331–1334, 1995.7.
3. Grace JN, Rand JA. Patellar instability after total knee arthroplasty. Clin Orthop 237:184–189, 1988.
4. Martin JW, Whiteside LA: The influence of joint line position on knee stability after condylar knee arthroplasty. Clin Orthop 259:146–156, 1990.
5. Whiteside LA, Summers RG: Anatomical landmarks for an intramedullary alignment system for total knee replacement. Orthop Trans 7:546–547, 1983.
6. Whiteside LA, Summers RG: The effect of the level of distal femoral resection on ligament balance in total knee replacement. In Dorr LD (ed). The Knee: Papers of the First Scientific Meeting of the Knee Society. Baltimore, University Park Press 59–73, 1984.
7. Whiteside LA, Kasselt MR, Haynes DW: Varus-valgus and rotational stability in rotationally unconstrained total knee arthroplasty. Clin Orthop 219:147–157, 1987.
8. Whiteside LA, McCarthy DS: Laboratory evaluation of alignment and kinematics in a unicompartmental knee arthroplasty inserted with intramedullary instrumentation. Clin Orthop 274:238–247, 1992.
9. Whiteside LA, Arima J: The anterior-posterior axis for femoral rotational alignment in valgus total knee arthroplasty. Clin Orthop 321:168–172, 1995.
10. Whiteside LA. Distal realignment of the patellar tendon to correct patellar tracking abnormalities in total knee arthroplasty. Clin Orthop 344:284–289, 1997.

Posterior Cruciate Ligament

3. Posterior Cruciate Ligament

Basic Principles

The posterior cruciate ligament serves a complex purpose throughout the entire flexion arc, acting primarily to prevent posterior travel of the tibia, but also performing secondary varus, valgus and rotational stabilizing roles when the collateral ligaments are deficient. It also provides resistance to hyperextension when the posterior capsule is deficient. Because the posterior cruciate ligament is a medial structure attached to the medial femoral condyle, it often contracts in the varus knee and stretches in the valgus knee. When it is contracted it often can be released partially, and much of its function can be preserved. Even when it is insufficient to provide adequate posterior stability, it can provide rotational and varus-valgus stabilization.

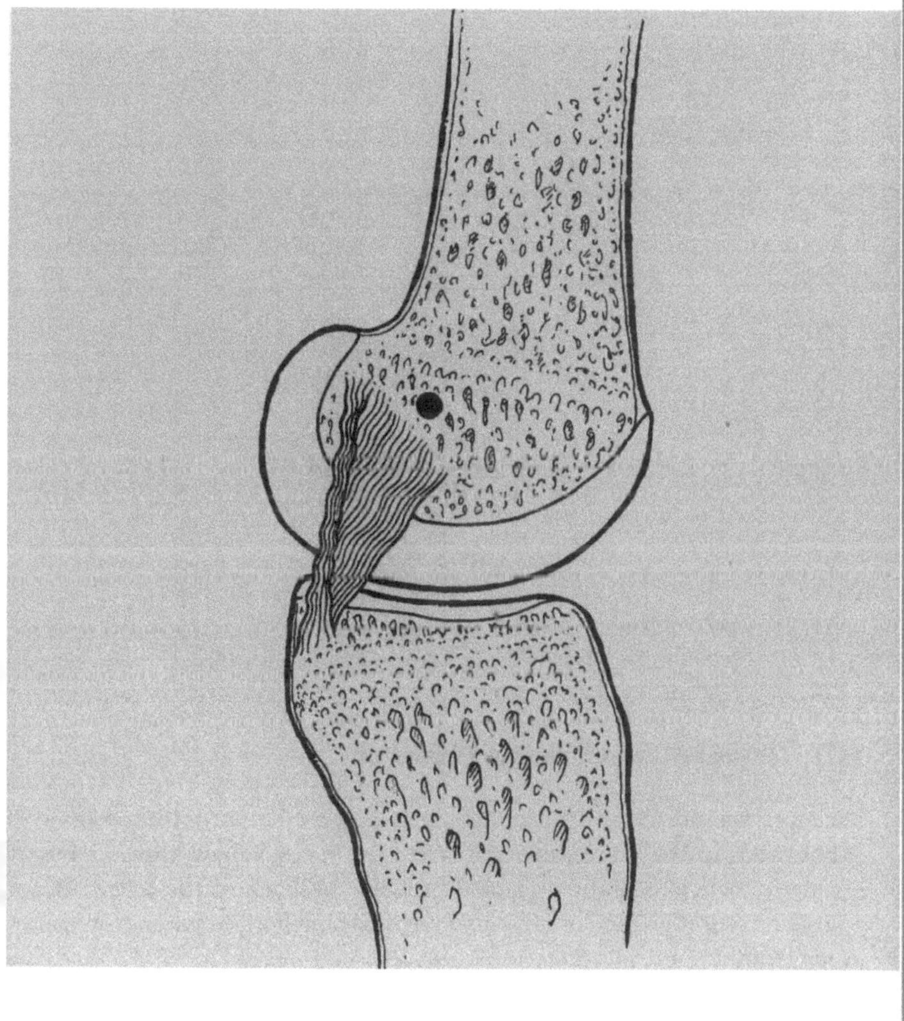

Fig. 32. The posterior cruciate ligament, like the medial collateral ligament, is attached over a broad band, so its anterior and posterior portions behave differently in flexion and extension. The anterior portion of the posterior cruciate ligament is attached to the femur distal to the epicondylar axis so it tends to loosen in full extension. The posterior portion, being behind the center of rotation, tends to tighten in hyper-extension. Both bands are relatively loose at 0° knee flexion.

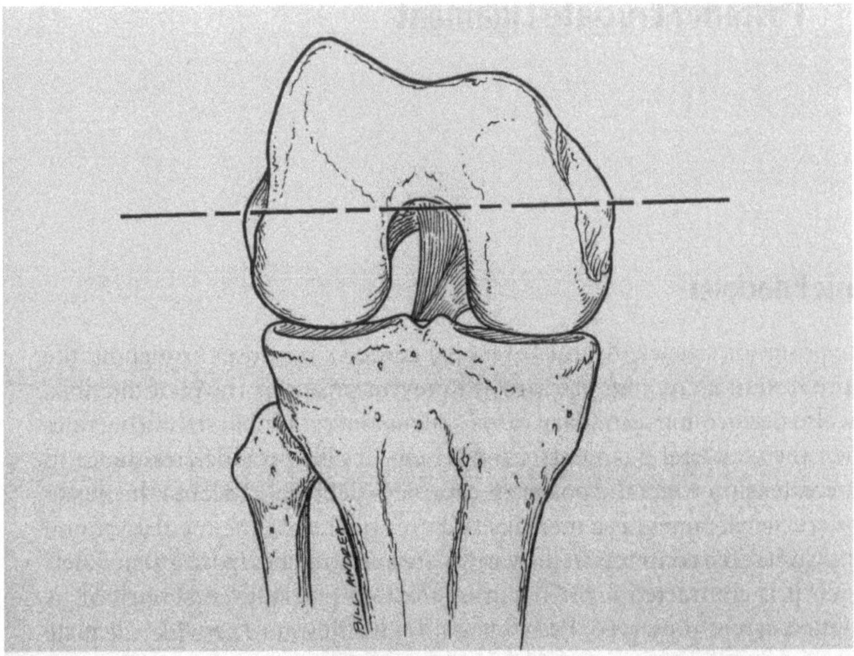

Fig. 33. In the flexed position, the anterolateral fibers are brought to tension and the posteromedial fibers loosen.

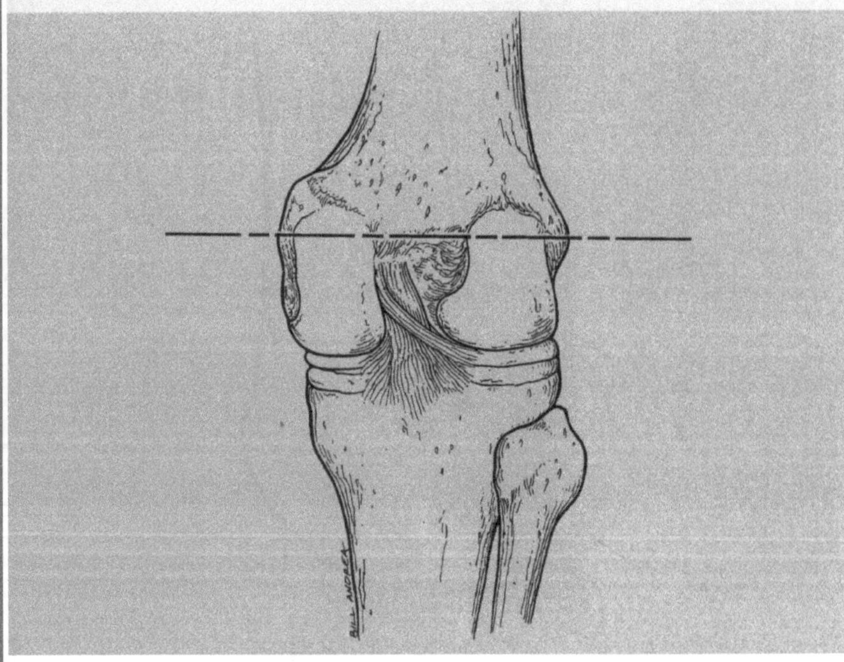

Fig. 34. Because the posterior cruciate ligament is attached to the medial femoral condyle, it tends to shorten in the varus knee and loosen in the valgus knee. The posterior cruciate ligament has auxillary attachments to the posterior portions of the menisci and joint capsule.

3.1. Tight Posterior Cruciate Ligament

Because the posterior cruciate ligament is a medial structure, it often is contracted in the varus knee and stretched in the valgus knee. The tight posterior cruciate ligament causes excessive rollback of the femur. When palpated with the knee in flexion, it feels extremely tight when it is abnormally tight.

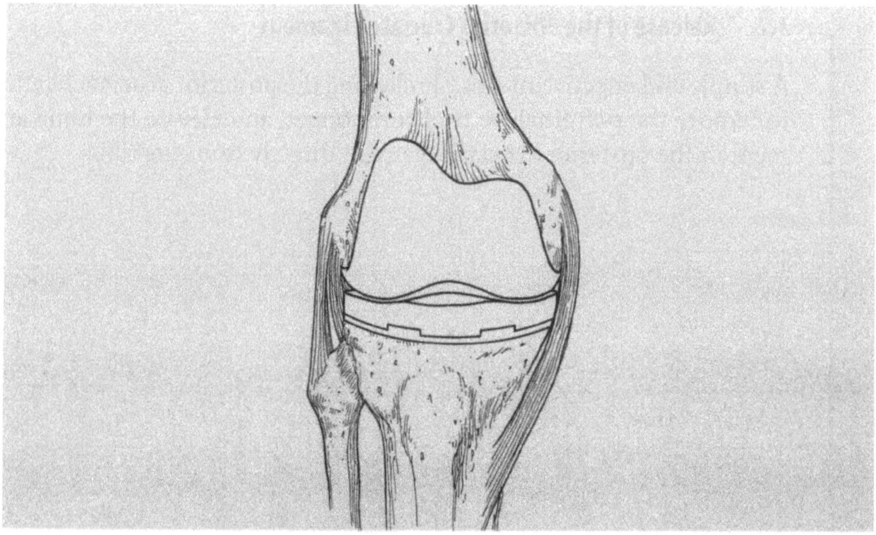

Fig. 35. The knee has normal stability in extension.

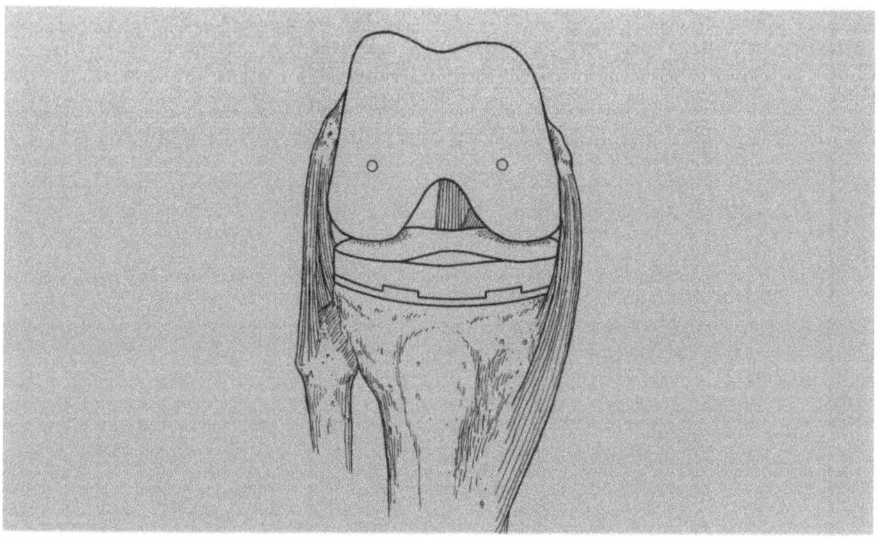

Fig. 36. But in flexion the femur rolls excessively posteriorly, and the posterior cruciate ligament is palpably tight. Neither collateral ligament is tight.

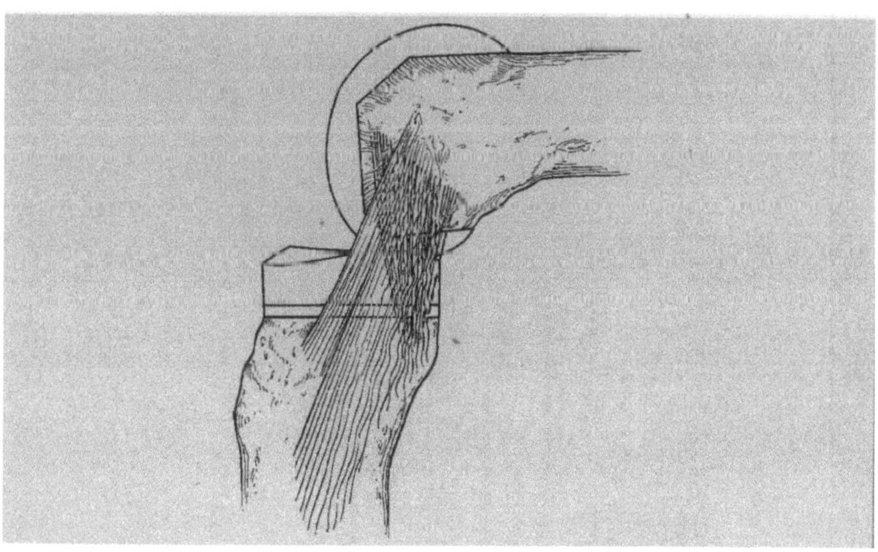

Fig. 37. On the side view, the femoral component is rolled excessively posteriorly, and is perched on the posterior edge of the tibial component. The anterior band of the medial collateral ligament also may be affected by this posterior position, and may seem to be excessively tight. The anterolateral portion of the posterior cruciate ligament is primarily responsible for the excessive posterior rollback.

3.2. Release of the Posterior Cruciate Ligament

A simple and effective means of releasing the posterior cruciate ligament is to remove the polyethylene trial component, and elevate the bone attachment of the posterior cruciate ligament directly from the tibia.

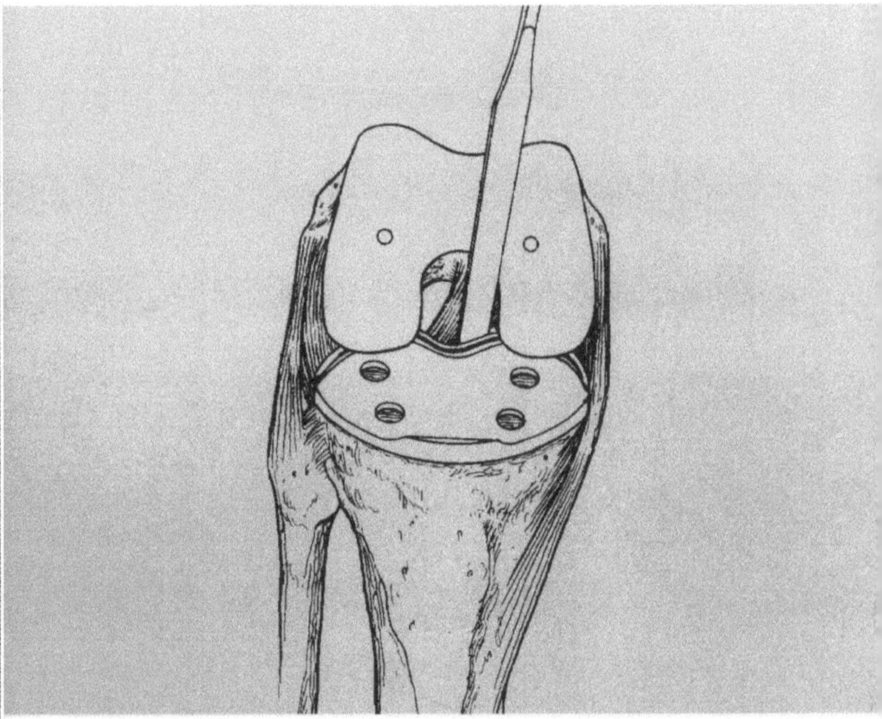

Fig. 38. The posterior cruciate ligament is released with a small segment of bone from its posterior tibial attachment. A quarter-inch osteotome is used to make several small cuts around the posterior cortical margin, and then the bone piece is levered loose.

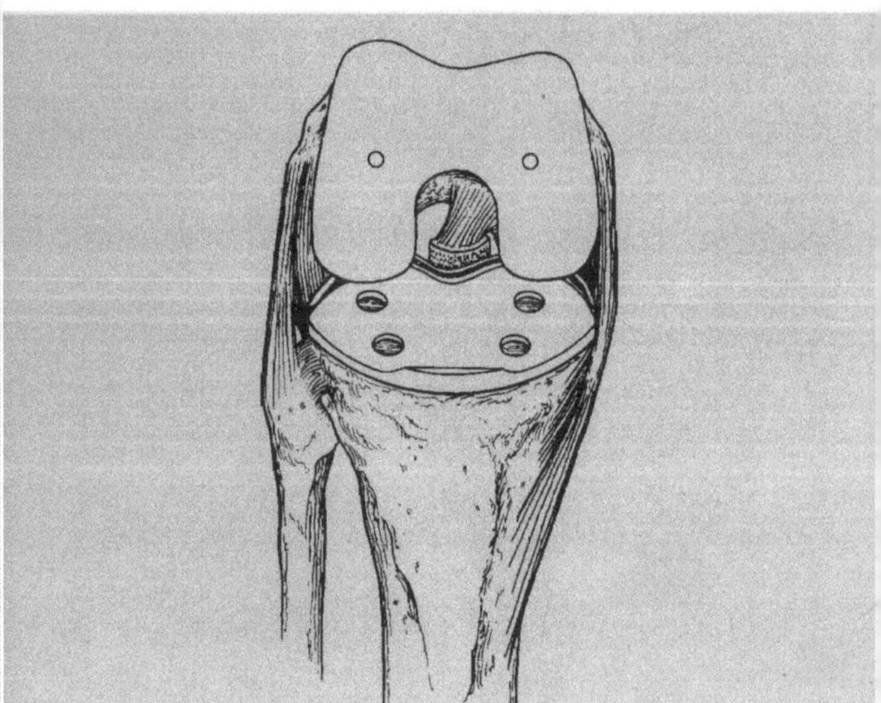

Fig. 39. The bone piece slides proximally 0.5cm–1cm, slackening the posterior cruciate ligament. The synovial membrane remains intact, and the ligament remains unfrayed by the release.

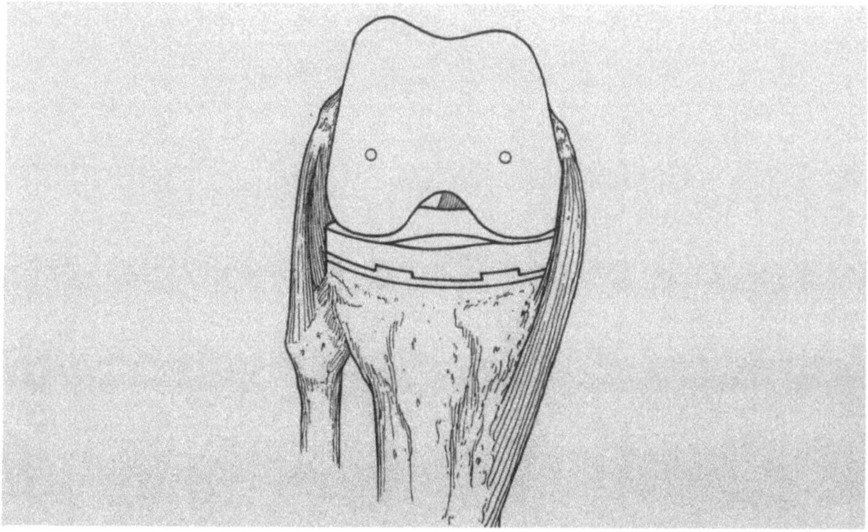

Fig. 40. After posterior cruciate ligament release the tibia slides posteriorly, and the femoral surfaces seat in the normal position on the tibial surfaces.

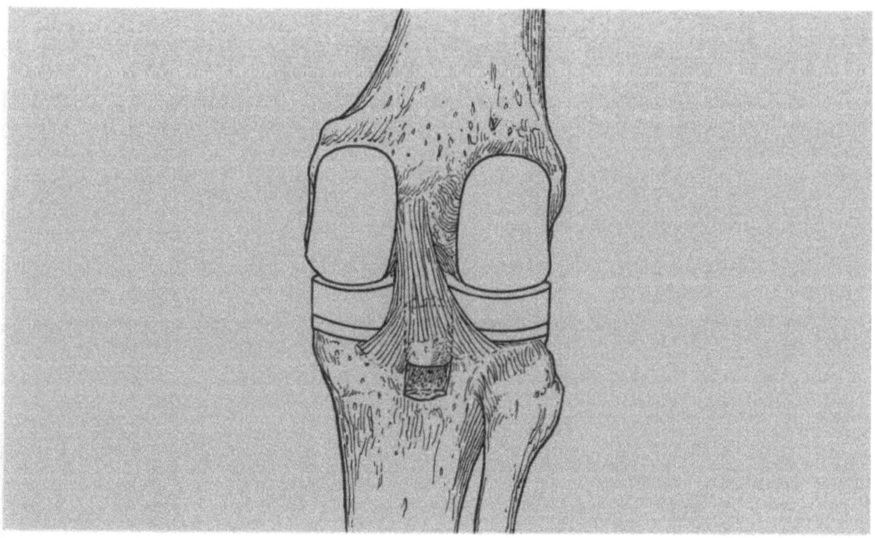

Fig. 41. The attachment of the posterior cruciate ligament has slid proximally, slackening the posterior cruciate ligament, but tightening the surrounding attachments of the posterior cruciate ligament so that they prevent excessive laxity.

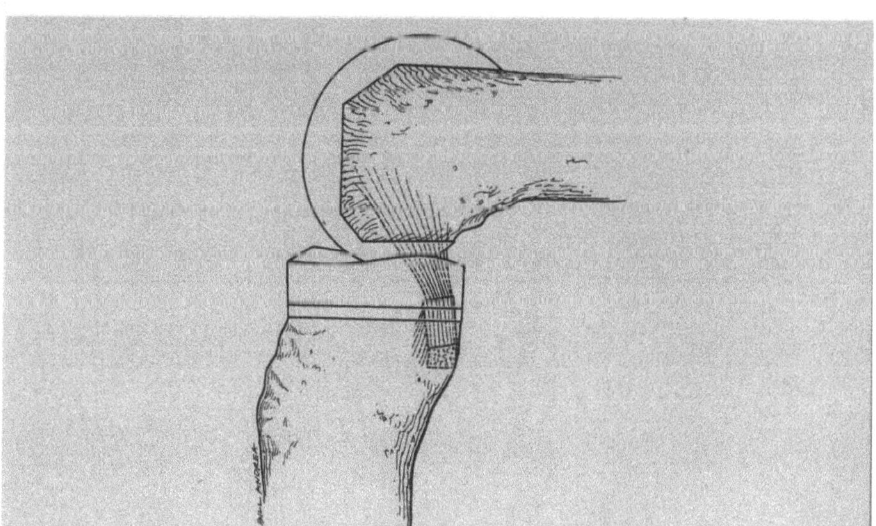

Fig. 42. The posterior cruciate ligament, in its new position, allows the tibia to slide posteriorly so that the femoral surfaces sit farther forward on the tibia.

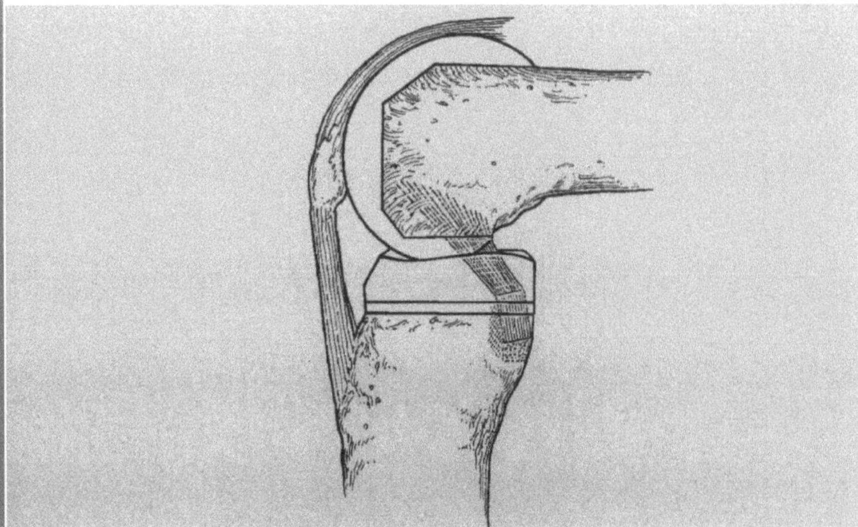

Fig. 43. After recession the posterior cruciate ligament, occasionally is elongated too much and the secondary posterior stabilizing structures are insufficient to prevent posterior sag. The femoral condyles seat far forward on the tibial surfaces and the tibia sags posteriorly. The quadriceps complex is placed at a disad-van-tage by this tibial position.

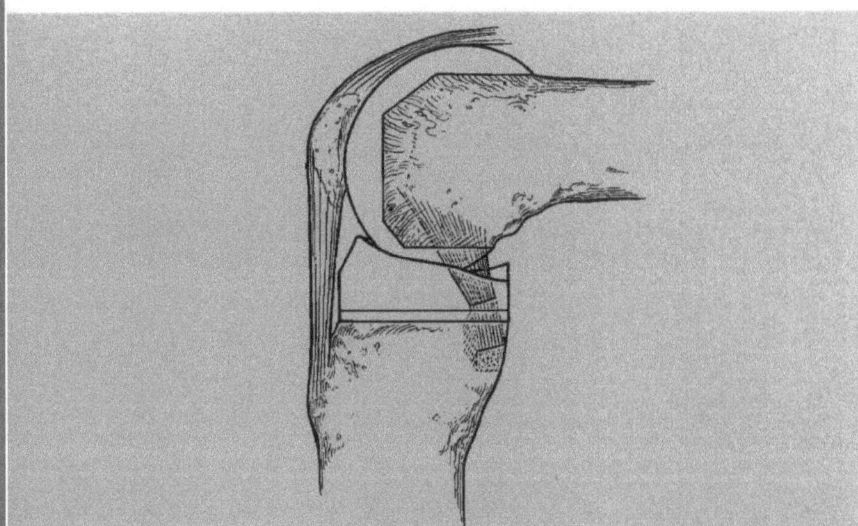

Fig. 44. When the conforming plus polyethylene insert is applied, posterior sag is controlled, and the tibia is held forward, improving the mechanical advantages of the quadriceps. The barrier to anterior dislocation of the femur is large both vertically and horizontally.

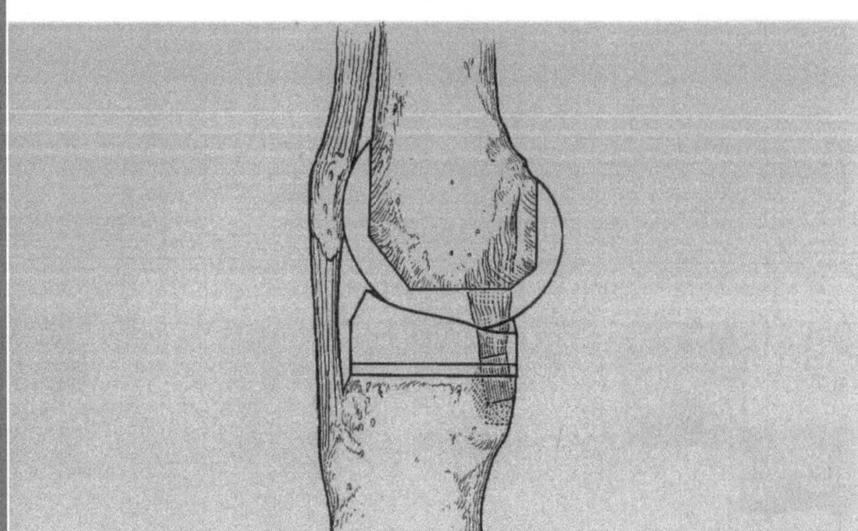

Fig. 45. In full extension the vertical and horizontal distance of travel required for subluxation also is large, and the tibia is held anteriorly by the anterior wall of the conforming plus prosthesis.

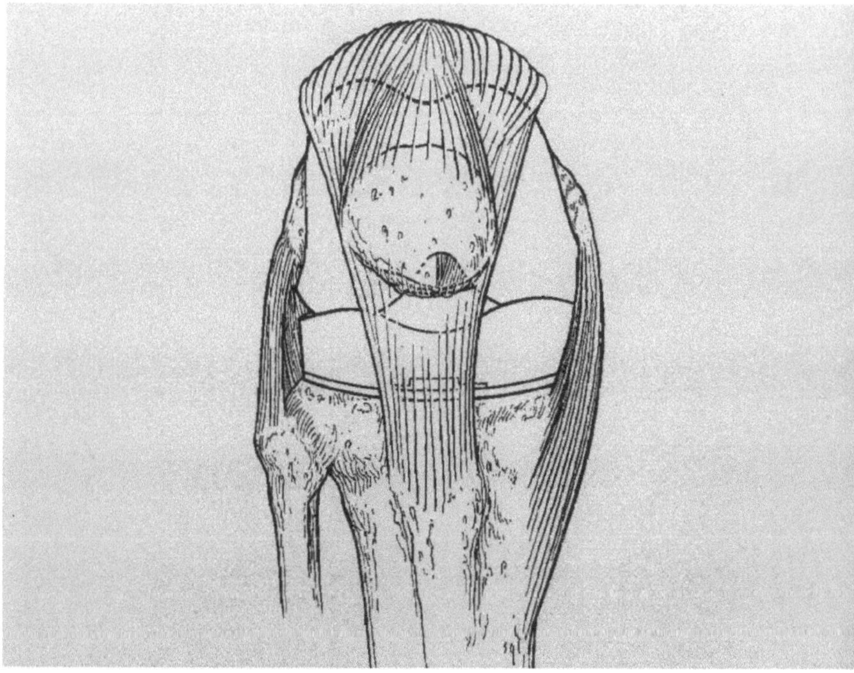

Fig. 46. When the patella is low, impingement against the anterior lip of the constrained polyethylene component is likely. In most cases these conforming-plus components are made with a recessed area for the patella.

Suggested Readings

1. Arima J, Whiteside LA, Martin JW, Miura H, White SE, McCarthy DS: Effect of partial release of the posterior cruciate ligament in total knee arthroplasty. Clin Orthop 353:194–202, 1998.
2. Hagena FW, Hofmann GO, Mittelmeier T, Wasmer G, Bergmann M: The cruciate ligament in knee replacement. Int Orthop 13:13–16, 1989.
3. Hughston JC: The posterior cruciate ligament in knee-joint stability. In: Proceedings of The American Academy of Orthopaedic Surgeons. J Bone Joint Surg Am 51:1045, 1969.
4. Lew WD, Lewis JL: The effect of knee-prosthesis geometry on cruciate ligament mechanics during flexion. J Bone Joint Surg Am 64:734–739, 1982.
5. Shoemaker SC, Daniel DM: The limits of knee motion. In Daniel DM, Akeson WH, O'Connor JJ (eds). Knee Ligaments. Structures, Function, Injury, and Repair. New York, Raven Press 153–161, 1990.

Varus Knee

4. Varus Knee

Basic Principles

Medial stability of the knee is a complex issue, and involves ligaments that behave differently in flexion and extension. The contracture and stretching that occur due to deformity and osteophytes affect these ligament structures unequally, and often cause different degrees of tightness or laxity in flexion and extension after the bone surfaces are resected correctly for varus-valgus alignment. The distortion of the joint surface also can cause varus-valgus alignment to differ in the flexed and extended positions, and the knee thus may require adjustment of portions of the medial stabilizing complex that affect stability either in flexion or extension.

The cornerstone of correct ligament balancing is correct varus-valgus alignment in flexion and extension. For alignment in the extended position, fixed anatomic landmarks such as the intramedullary canal of the femur and long axis of the tibia are accepted. When the joint surface is resected at an angle of 5° to 7° valgus to the medullary canal of the femur and perpendicular to the long axis of the tibia, the joint surfaces are perpendicular to the mechanical axis of the lower extremity, and roughly parallel to the epicondylar axis in the extended position. In the flexed position, anatomic landmarks are equally important for varus-valgus alignment. Incorrect varus-valgus alignment in flexion not only malaligns the long axes of the femur and tibia, but also incorrectly positions the patellar groove both in flexion and extension. Finding suitable landmarks for varus-valgus alignment has led to efforts to use the posterior femoral condyles, epicondylar axis, and anterior-posterior axis of the femur. The posterior femoral condyles provide excellent rotational alignment landmarks if the femoral joint surface has not been worn or otherwise distorted by developmental abnormalities or the arthritic process. However, as with the distal surfaces, the posterior femoral condylar surfaces sometimes are damaged or hypoplastic (more commonly in the valgus than in the varus knee) and cannot serve as reliable anatomic guides for alignment. The epicondylar axis is anatomically inconsistent and in all cases other than revision total knee arthroplasty with severe bone loss, is unreliable for varus-valgus alignment in flexion just as it is in extension. The anterior-posterior axis, defined by the center of the intercondylar notch posteriorly and the deepest part of the patellar groove anteriorly, is highly consistent, and always lies within the median sagittal plane that bisects the lower extremity, passing through the hip, knee, and ankle. When the articular surfaces are resected perpendicular to the anterior-posterior axis, they are perpendicular to the anterior-posterior plane, and the extremity can function normally in this plane throughout the arc of flexion.

In the presence of articular surface deformity the anatomic references are especially important for correct varus-valgus alignment. The usual reliable landmarks for varus-valgus alignment of the femoral component in flexion include the posterior femoral condyles, the long axis of the tibia, and the tensed supporting ligaments. If the posterior femoral condyle wears and the tibial plateau collapses on the medial side of the knee, these normally reliable landmarks cannot be used. Instead, the anterior-posterior axis of the femur is used as a reference line for the femoral cuts and the long axis of the tibia is used for a reference line for the tibial cut so that the joint surfaces are cut perpendicular to these two reference lines. Once the joint surfaces have been resected correctly to establish normal varus-valgus alignment in flexion and extension, the trial com-ponents are inserted and ligament function is assessed in flexion and extension. The "liga-ments are released according to their function at each position. The medial collateral ligament (deep and superficial layers) attaches to the medial epicondylar area through a broad band. The posterior oblique portion, which spreads posteriorly over the medial tibial flare and incorporates the sheath of the semimembranosus tendon, tightens in extension. The anterior portion of the ligament complex, which extends anteriorly along the medial tibial flare, tightens in flexion and loosens in extension. The posterior capsule is loose in flexion, and tightens only in full extension. With this information the medial ligament structures of the knee can be released individually according to the position in which excessive tightness is found.

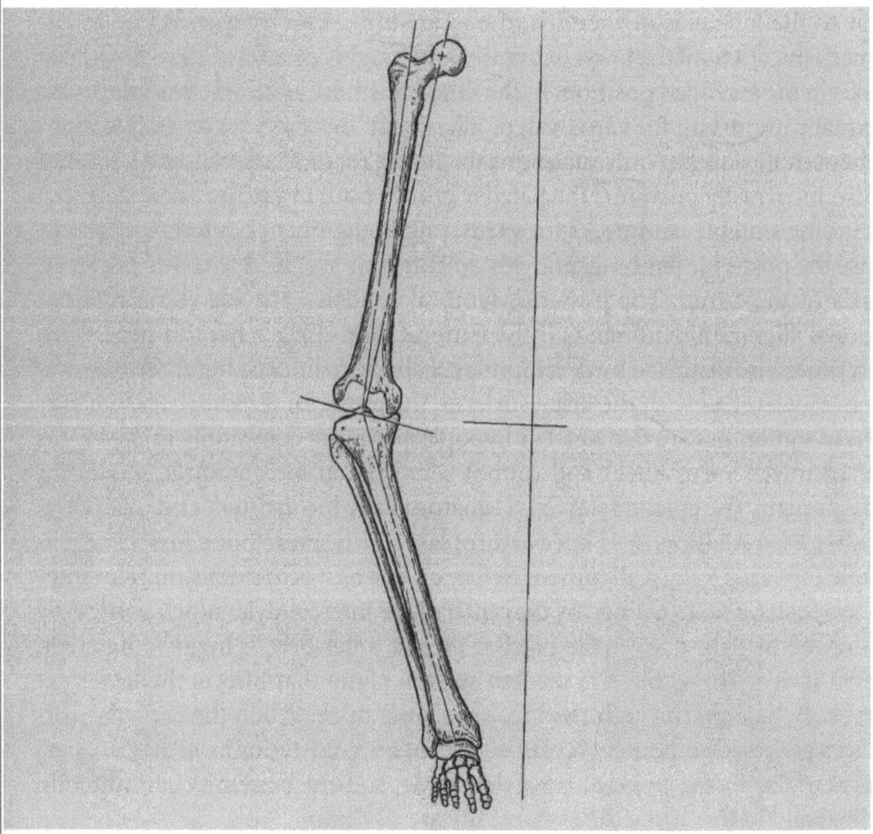

Fig. 47. In the varus knee the femoral condyles are configured normally, and a line through the long axis of the femoral diaphysis crosses the joint line in the center of the patellar groove. The varus malalignment of the extremity is caused by a defect in the medial tibial plateau. A line through the center of the tibial diaphysis crosses the joint in the center of the notch between the tibial spines. Entry points into the joint for intramedullary alignment rods are made in the center of the patellar groove and directly between the tibial spines.

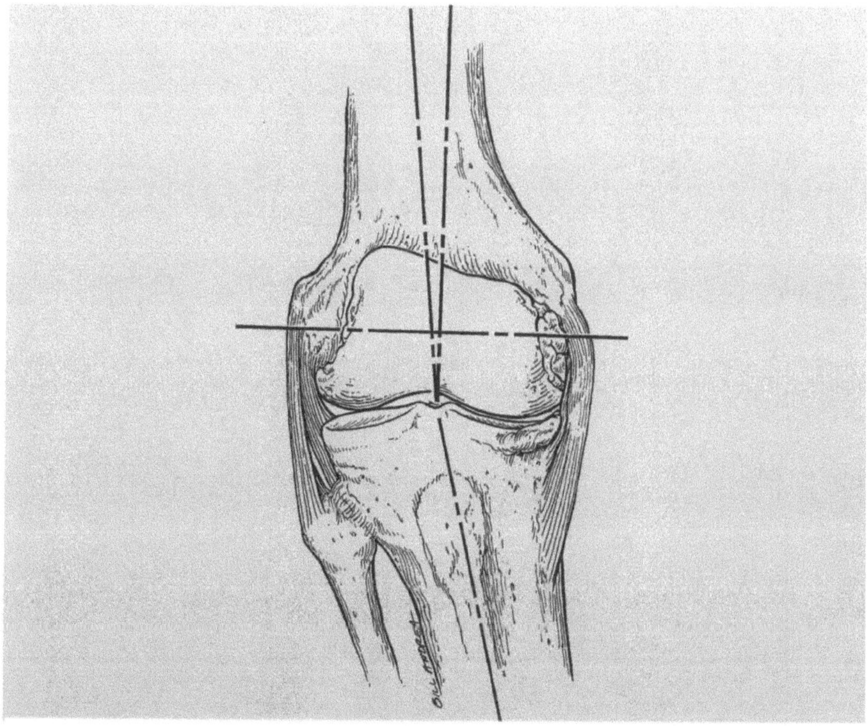

Fig. 48. The varus knee has a group of bone and ligament abnormalities that must be addressed to correct the deformity. The mechanical axis of the femur is tilted medially relative to the long axis of the tibia. The distal femoral surface usually remains in valgus alignment to the long axis of the femur. Most of the varus deformity is caused by deficiency in the medial tibial plateau. The deep and superficial medial collateral ligaments are contracted and deformed by osteophytes.

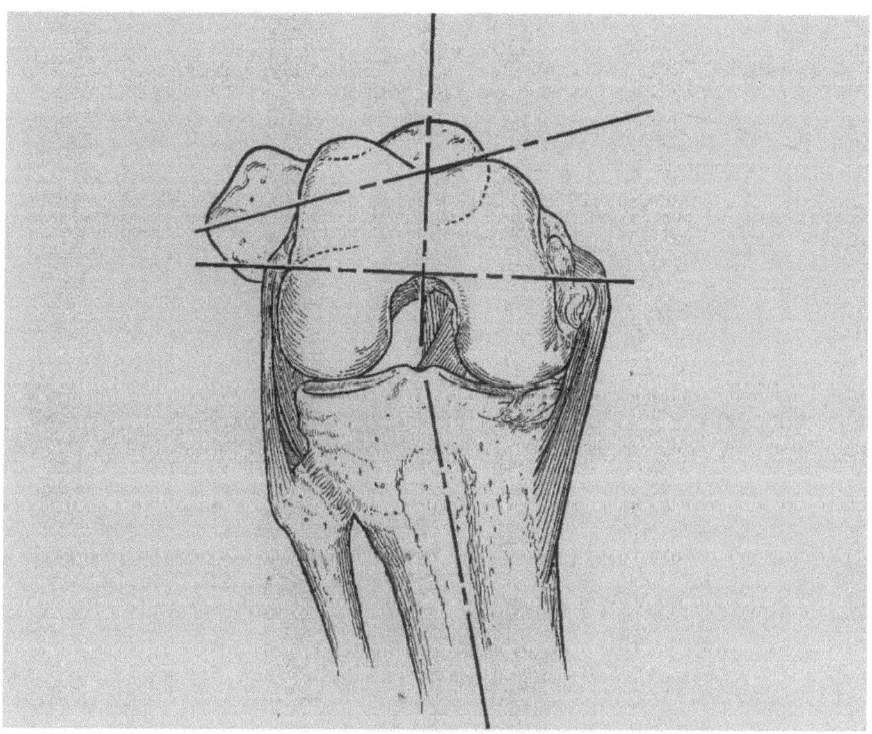

Fig. 49. In the flexed position the mechanical abnormalities are similar. The deficiency in the medial tibial plateau causes the tibia to tilt toward varus, and the anterior-posterior axis of the femur tilts medially relative to the long axis of the tibia. Here the hip is in neutral position with the anterior-posterior axis passing through the center of the femoral head, and the femoral neck anteverted 15° to the epicondylar axis. The deep and superficial medial collateral ligaments are contracted, and the posterior cruciate ligament, being a medial structure, often is contracted as well.

Finding the anterior-posterior axis can be difficult if the intercondylar notch is distorted by osteophytes. However, the lateral edge of the posterior cruciate ligament is consistently in the center of the intercondylar notch, and can usually be identified easily without remaining the osteophytes.

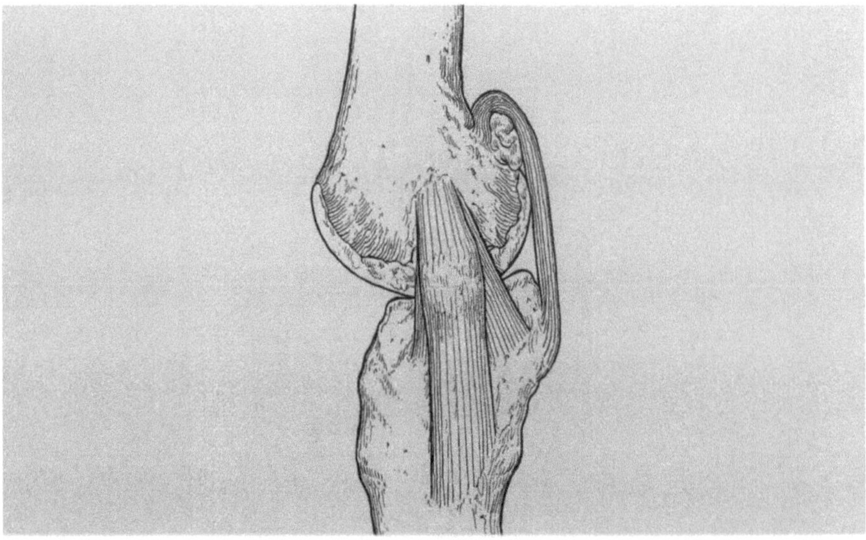

Fig. 50. The osteophytes may deform the medial collateral ligament and posterior capsule enough to cause flexion contracture.

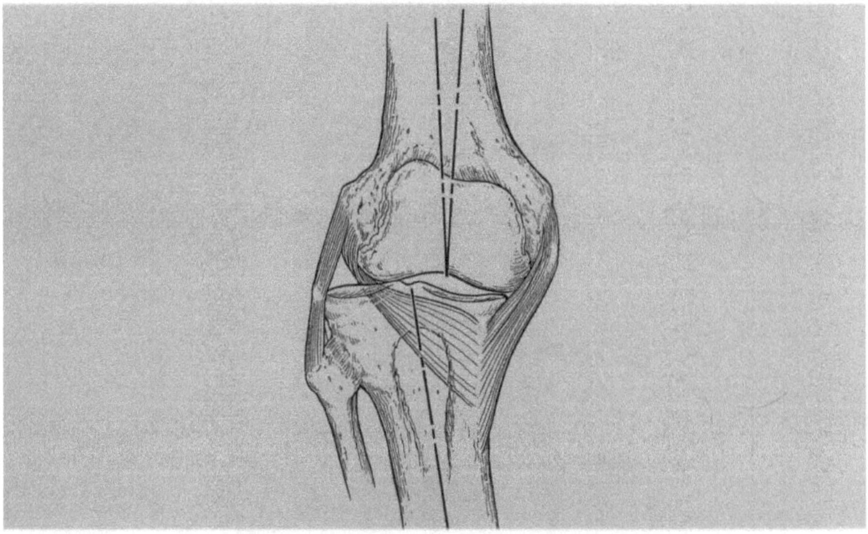

Fig. 51. The tibia often is subluxed laterally in the varus knee, shifting the origin of the popliteus muscle proximally and laterally, and shortening the popliteus complex.

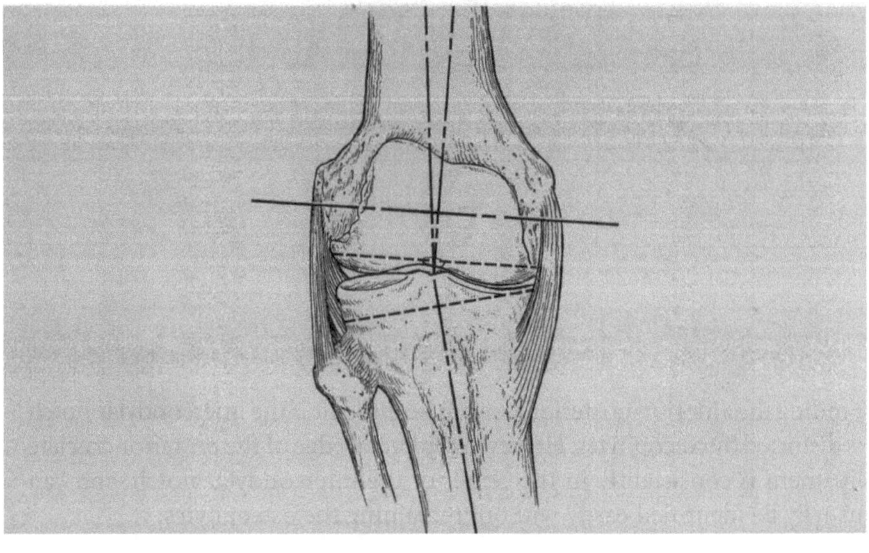

Fig. 52. The distal surfaces of the femur are resected perpendicular to the mechanical axis, which is approximately parallel to the epicondylar axis. This is facilitated by aligning the resection guide at 5° valgus to the long axis of the femur. Because deformity of the distal femoral joint surface is rare in the varus knee, approximately equal thickness of bone usually is resected from the medial and lateral sides. The upper surface of the tibia is resected perpendicular to the long axis of the tibia, resecting the thickness of the tibial component (10–12 mm) from the intact lateral side, and much less from the deficient medial tibial plateau. In many cases a defect is left in the medial tibial plateau.

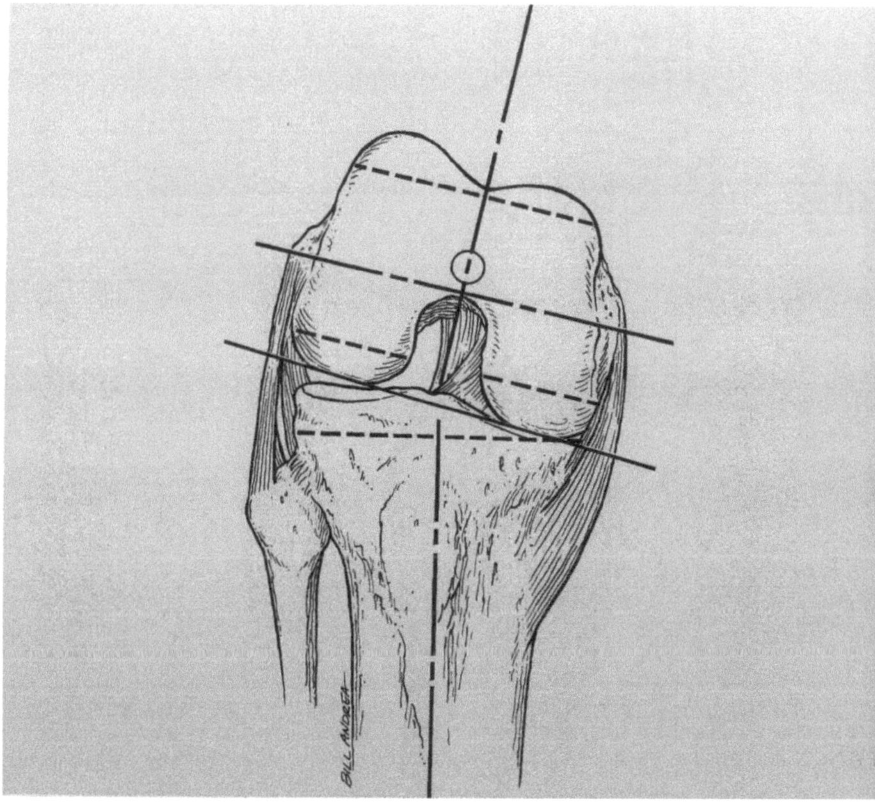

Fig. 53. The anterior and posterior surfaces of the femur are resected perpendicular to the anterior-posterior axis and parallel to the epicondylar axis. Similar to the long axis of the femur, the anterior-posterior axis is used as a reliable reference axis to align these cuts. This axis is identified by marking the lateral edge of the posterior cruciate ligament and the deepest part of the patellar groove. The articular surfaces are resected perpendicular to the anterior-posterior axis and parallel to the epicondylar axis. In most cases of varus knee the posterior femoral condyles maintain their normal 3° medial down-slope, and can be used for alignment of the femoral component in flexion. In this case, a 3° external rotational guide would be used to engage the posterior femoral condyles in order to place the anterior and posterior femoral surfaces in neutral alignment. The long axis of the tibia is used as a reference for the upper tibial resection. This surface is resected perpendicular to the tibial long axis when viewed from the front, and with a 4° to 7° posterior slope when viewed from the side.

The sequence in which the procedures are performed is important in total knee replacement. Resection of the femoral surfaces makes the tibial surfaces accessible. Resection of the tibial surface clears the way to remove the osteophytes. Removal of the osteophytes frees the ligaments so they may be assessed and released as needed. No ligament should be released until all the osteophytes are removed otherwise excessive laxity may occur. Extra bone should not be removed to correct a flexion contracture until all ligament balancing has been finished, otherwise inappropriate laxity in extension may occur once ligament release has been done.

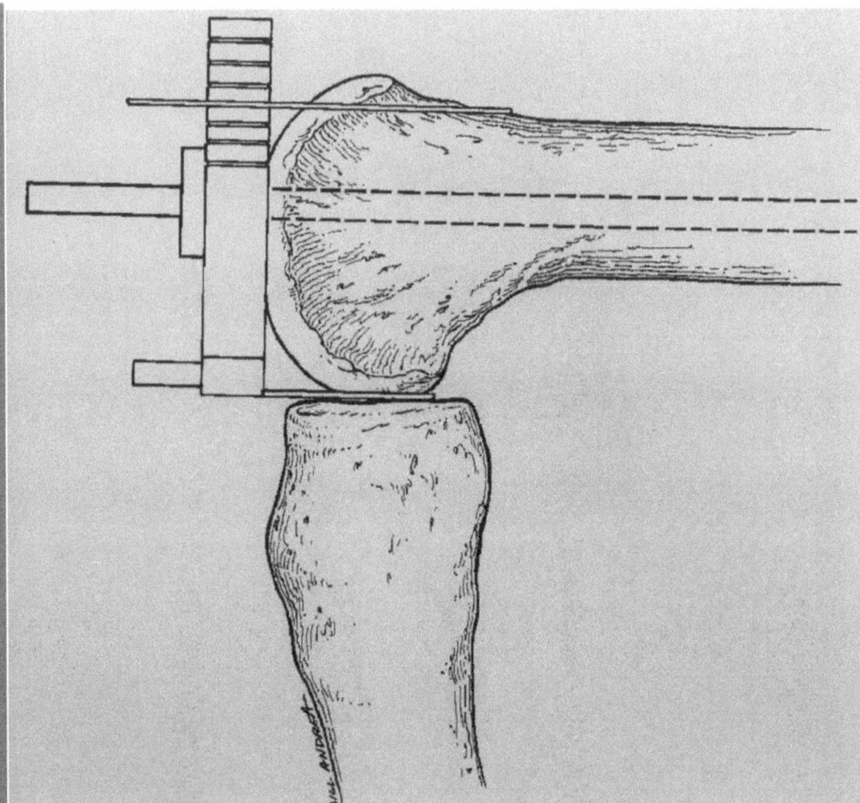

Fig. 54. The femur is sized from the anterior cortex (just proximal to the joint surface) to the posterior femoral joint surface. Resection guides are used to measure and remove the thickness of the implant from all intact surfaces of the femur. An anterior stylus is used to position the resection guide so that the anterior surface cut aligns flush with the anterior cortex of the femur. Posterior paddles are used to engage the posterior femoral condyles. These posterior paddles are used to confirm the anterior-posterior size of the femur and also to serve as a guide for rotational alignment (varus-valgus alignment in flexion) of the femoral component.

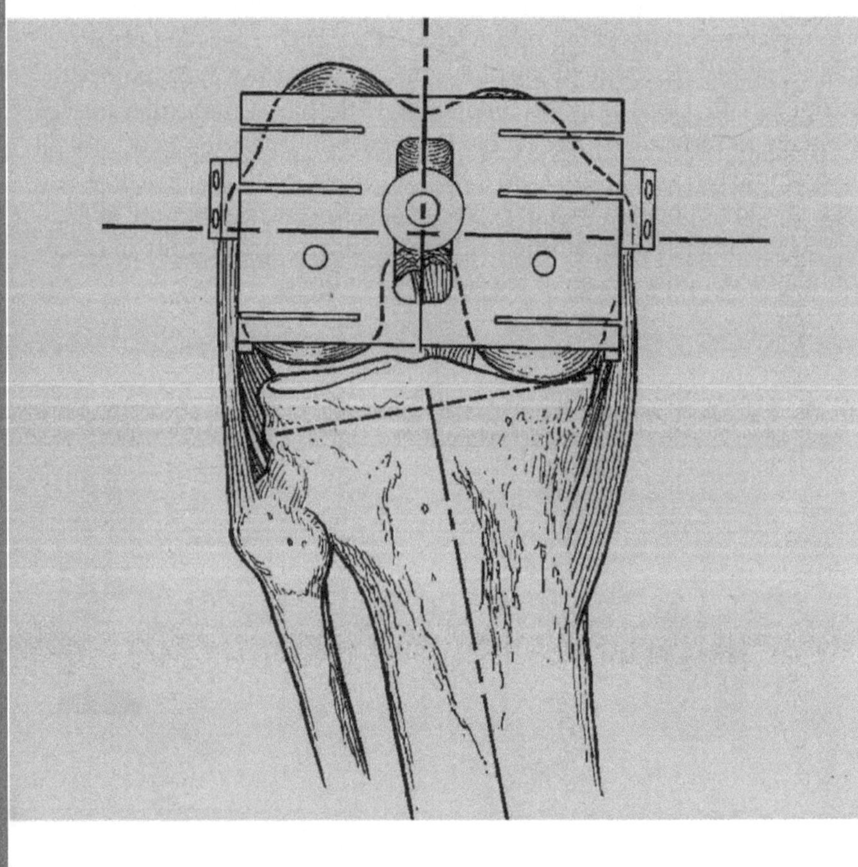

Fig. 55. Varus-valgus alignment of the femoral component in flexion (rotational alignment) is determined by the anterior-posterior axis. Here the cutting guide is aligned with the anterior-posterior axis of the femur. The anterior-posterior plane of the femur is defined by the lateral edge of the posterior cruciate ligament and the deepest point in the patellar groove. This also aligns the femoral surface cuts parallel to the epicondylar axis. Three degrees of external rotational alignment relative to the posterior femoral condylar surface would also achieve neutral varus-valgus alignment in this case since there is no posterior condylar surface deformity.

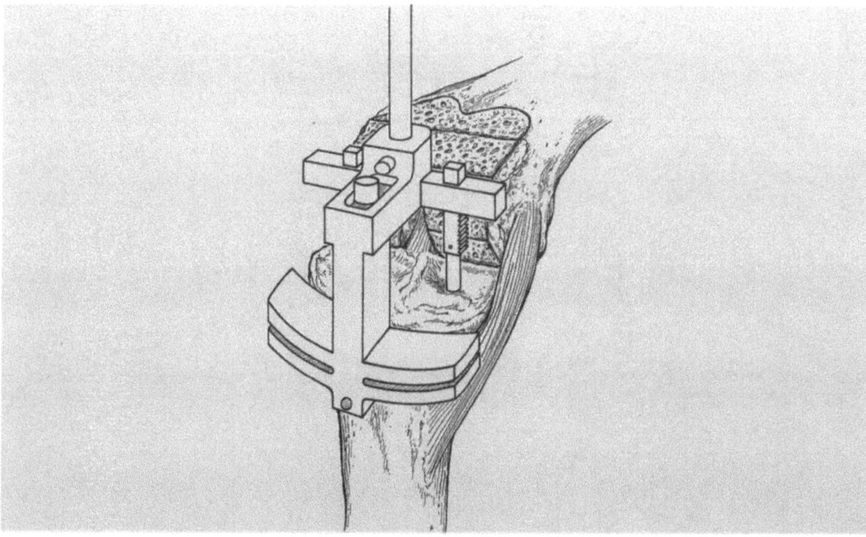

Fig. 56. After removal of all resected segments from the distal femoral surfaces, the tibial alignment instrument is applied and the upper surface of the tibia is resected. In most cases the tibial surface is resected perpendicular to the long axis of the tibia in the coronal plane, but it is sloped 4° to 7° posteriorly in the sagittal plane to match the normal slope of the tibia.

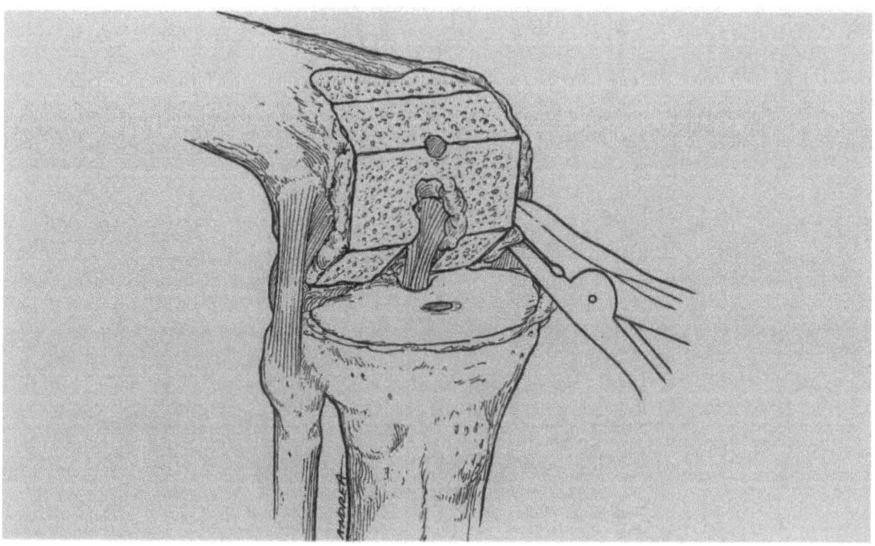

Fig. 57. After the tibial surface is removed, the osteophytes are first removed from the medial femoral edge anteriorly, distally, and then posteriorly, carefully teasing them from the deep medial collateral ligament.

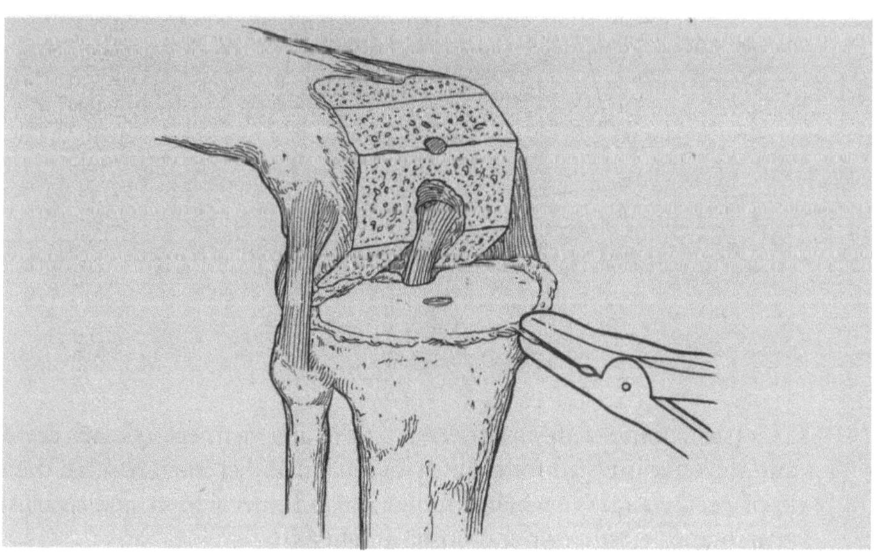

Fig. 58. Next the osteophytes are cleared from the intercondylar notch while care is taken to avoid damage to the posterior cruciate ligament. The medial tibial osteophyte is removed next, all the way around the posterior edge.

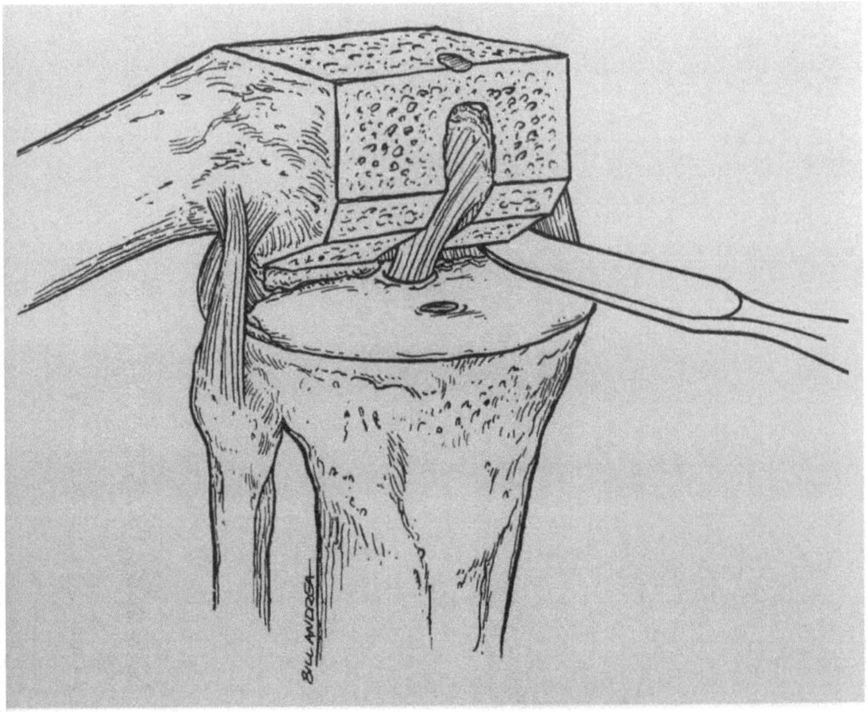

Fig. 59. After the medial tibial osteophyte has been removed, the knee will be freed enough to allow easy access to the posterior femoral osteophytes. They are cut free with a curved half-inch osteotome and the same osteotome is used to free the osteophyte in the popliteus recess laterally.

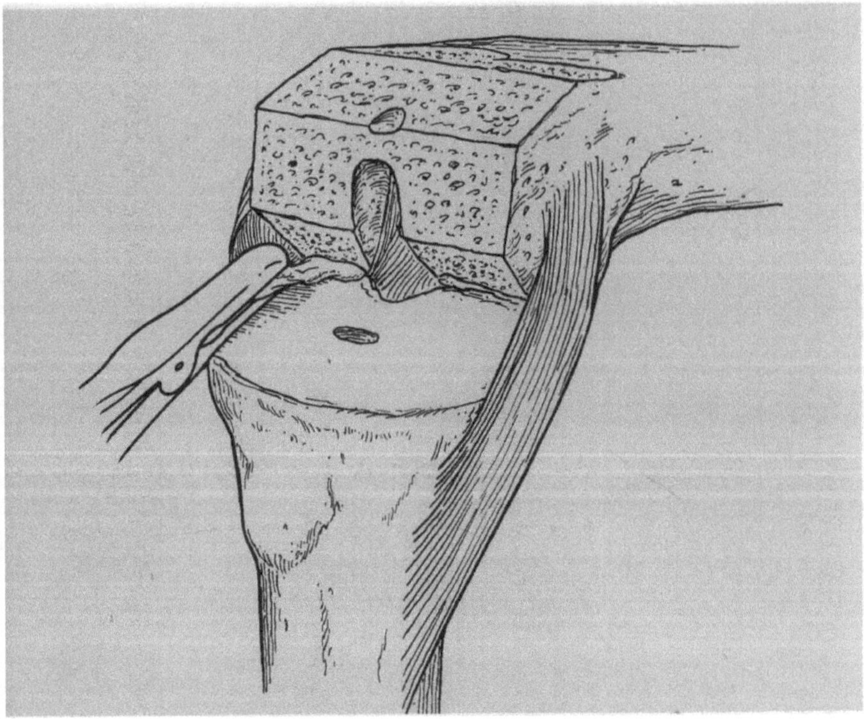

Fig. 60. Finally, the osteophytes are teased loose from the posterior capsule and the osteophyte that surrounds the popliteus tendon is removed from the popliteus recess.

The trial components are inserted before any ligament releases are done, and the knee is tested for stability in flexion and extension. With the trials in place, the knee is evaluated in flexion and extension to assess varus, valgus, rotational, anterior and posterior stability.

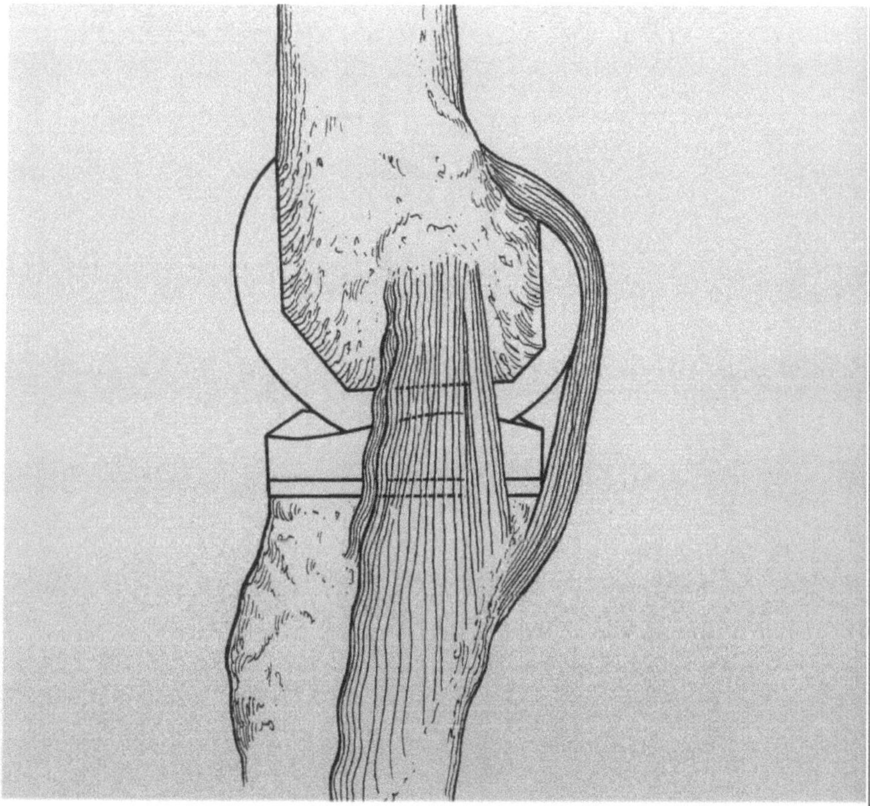

Fig. 61. The medial collateral ligament attaches to the medial femoral condyle over a fairly broad area, and this affects the function of the ligament in flexion and extension. With the knee fully extended, the posterior capsule and the posteromedial oblique portion of the medial collateral ligament are tight. The anterior portion of the medial collateral ligament loosens in full extension, but being close to the center of rotation, it acts as a stabilizing structure through-out the flexion-extension arc.

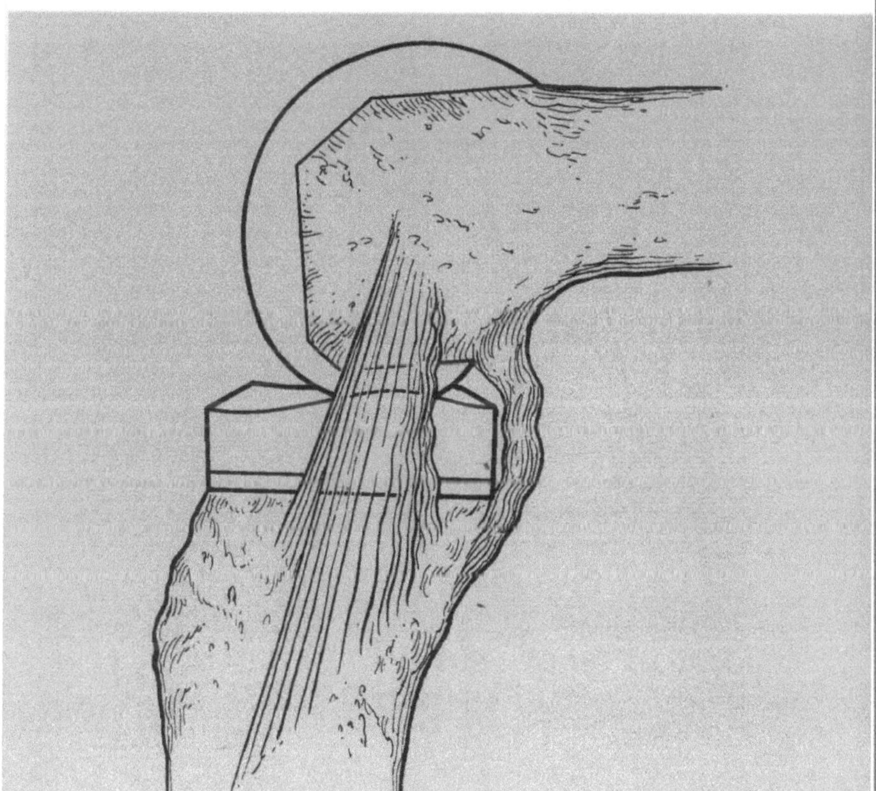

Fig. 62. When the knee flexes the posterior capsule and the postero-medial oblique portion of the medial collateral ligament loosen. The anterior portion of the medial collateral ligament tightens.

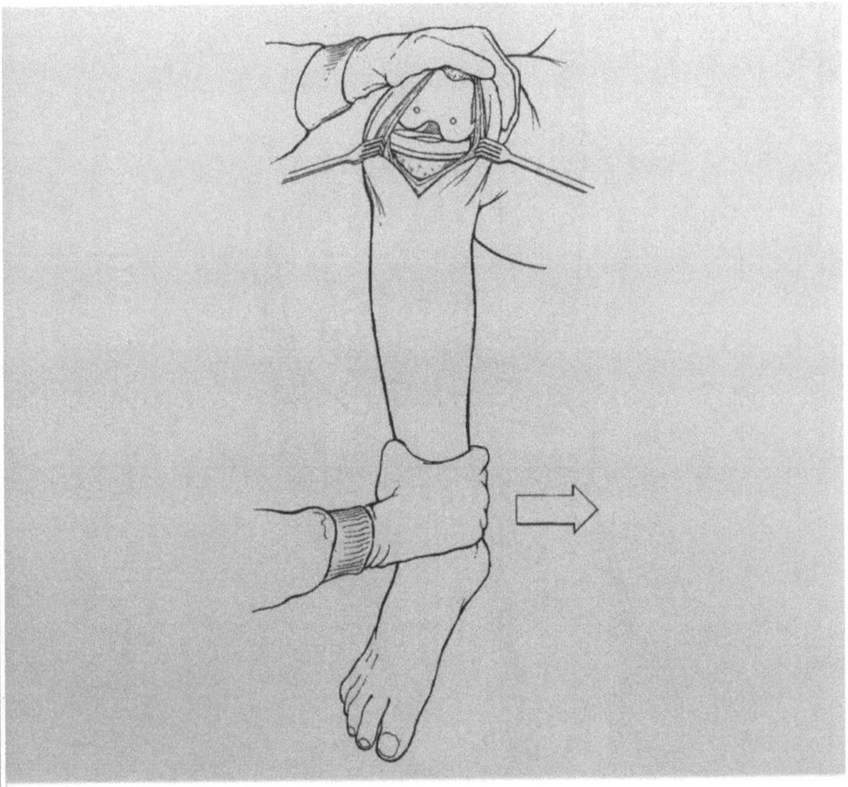

Fig. 63. To test the knee in flexion, the ankle is grasped with one hand while the other hand steadies the knee. The extremity then is rotated internally through the hip until the medial ligaments are stressed, then rotated externally until the lateral ligaments are stressed.

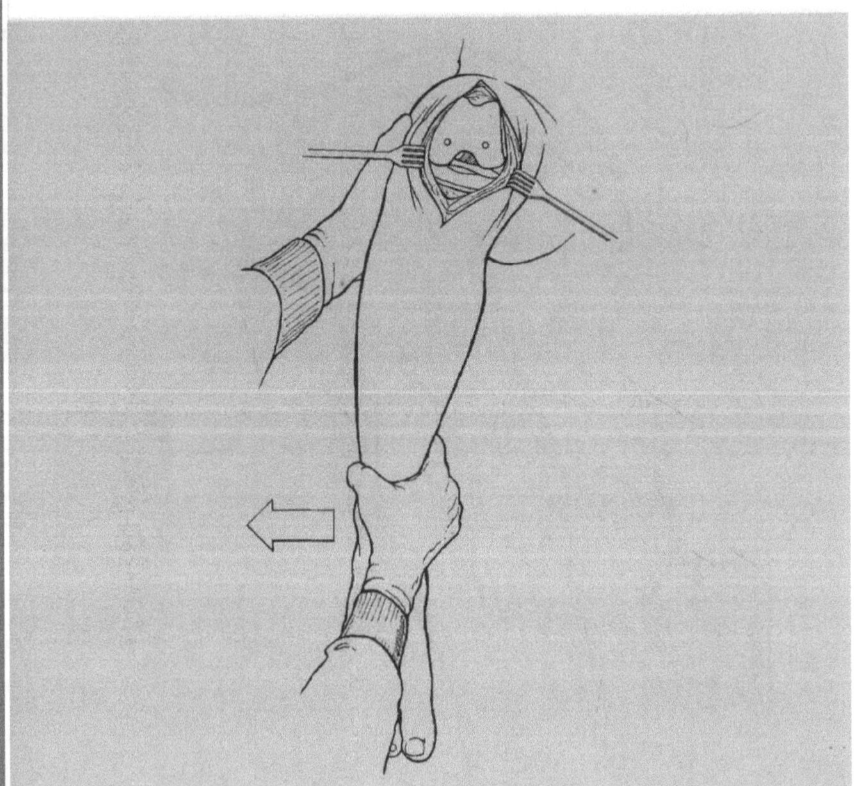

Fig. 64. The tibia is rotated to assess rotational stability, then the tibia is grasped just below the tibial tubercle and pushed posteriorly and pulled anteriorly to assess anterior-posterior stability.

4.1. Tight Medially in Flexion, Loose in Extension

In some cases the medial structures are not contracted uniformly, and the knee may be tight medially only in flexion, but not in extension.

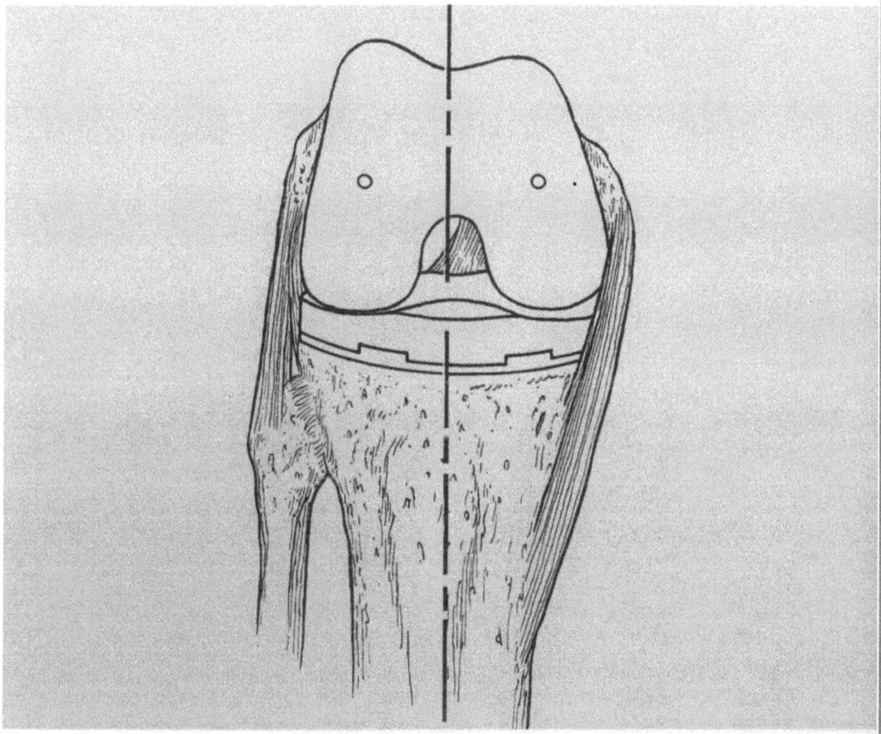

Fig. 65. The anterior portion of the medial collateral ligament is excessively tight in flexion. The medial femoral condyle sits further posteriorly than does the lateral femoral condyle and the tibia tends to pivot around the medial collateral ligament. Otherwise the knee is well aligned, and the anterior-posterior axis and long axis of the tibia align well with one another. The posterior cruciate ligament is soft to palpation, and is not a deforming structure.

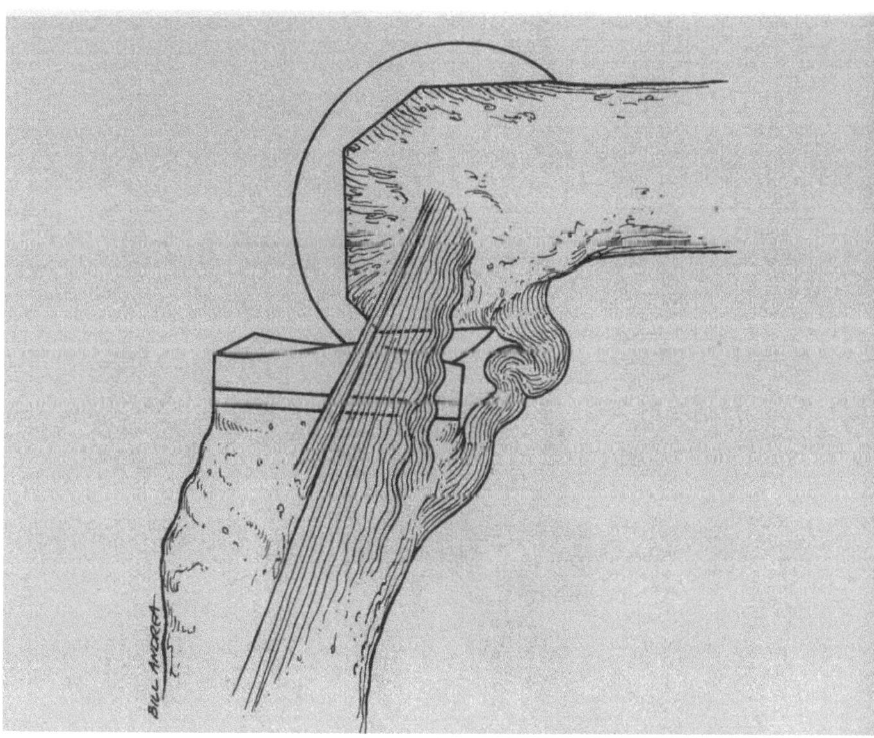

Fig. 66. The posterior portion of the medial collateral ligament is loose in flexion, and does not contribute to the ligament imbalance. The anterior portion is tight and definitely contributes to the ligament imbalance.

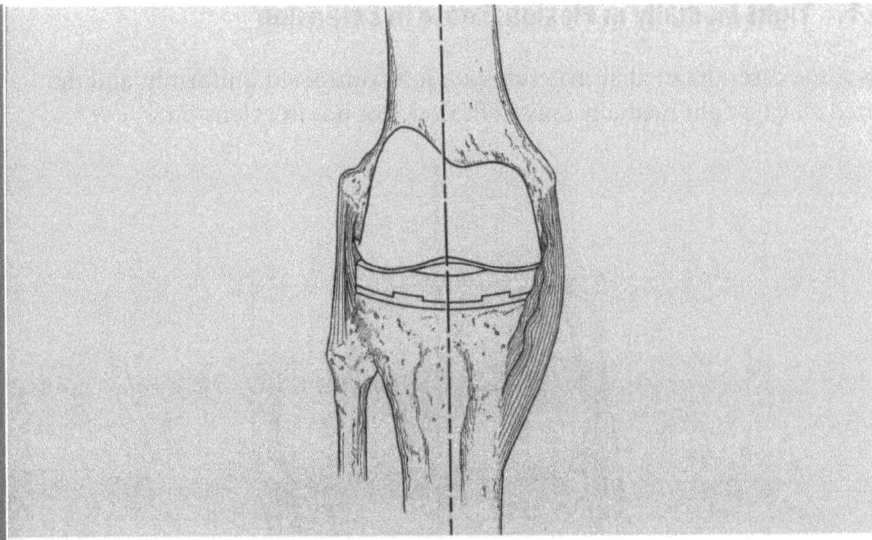

Fig. 67. In extension the anterior portion of the medial collateral ligament slackens normally, so ligament balance is normal in extension.

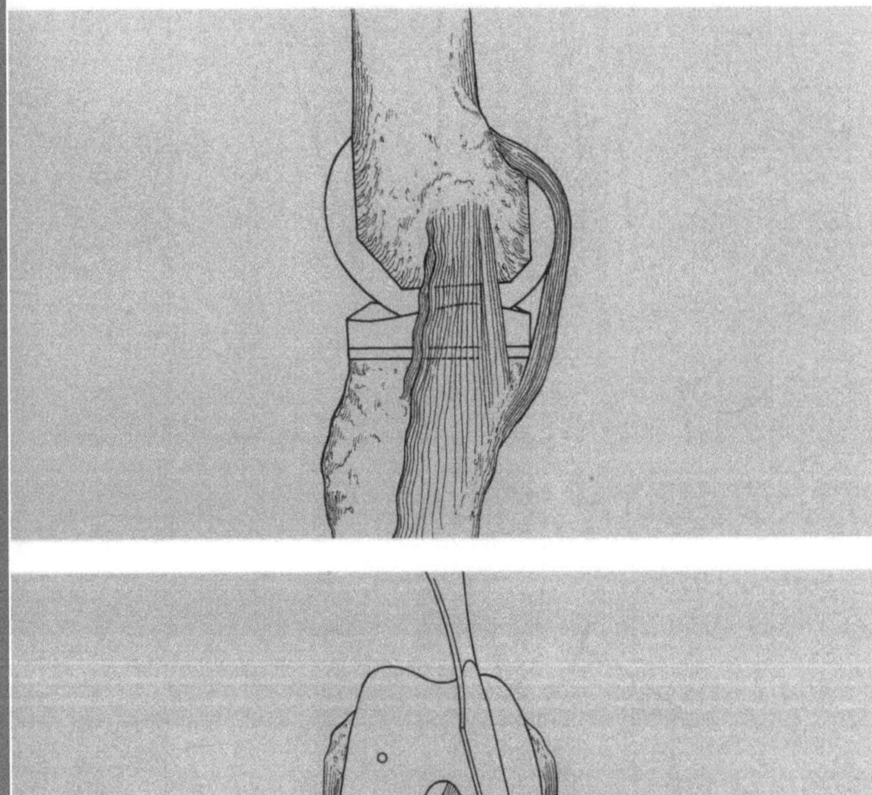

Fig. 68. The posterior portion of the medial collateral ligament becomes taught in extension, and the anterior portion slackens so that the knee has normal ligament balance in extension.

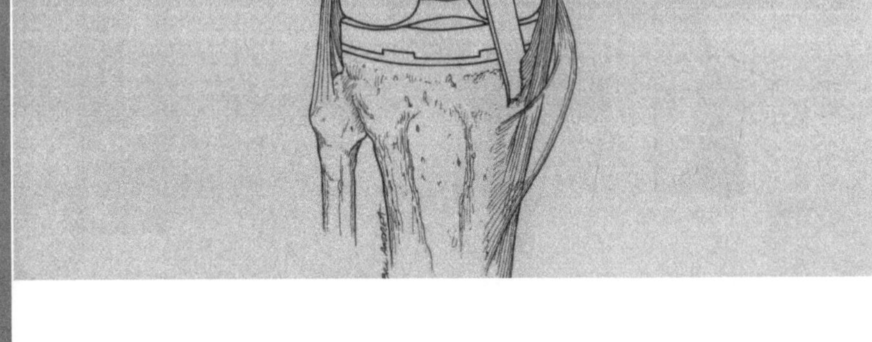

Fig. 69. This imbalance is corrected by releasing the anterior portion of the medial collateral ligament. The knee is flexed to 90° and a curved 1/2-inch osteotome is used to elevate the anterior portion of the deep and superficial medial collateral ligament subperiosteally while leaving the attachment of the pes anserinus intact.

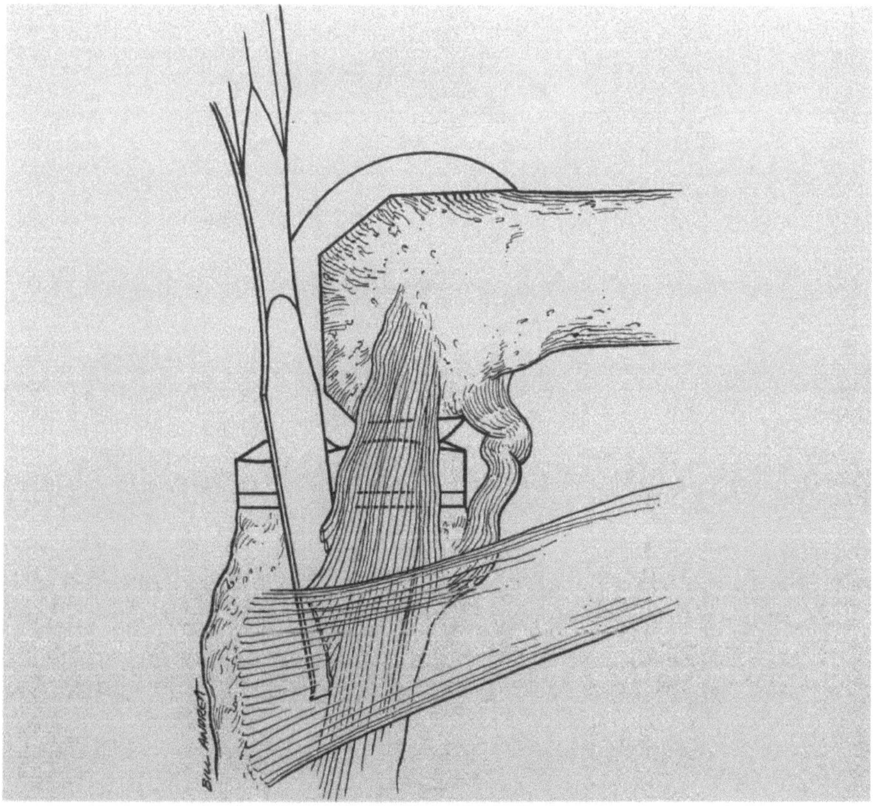

Fig. 70. The taught anterior fibers are released subperiosteally. These fibers attach fairly far distally (8–10 cm), and the osteotome is passed far enough to completely release the anterior fibers. The attachment of the pes anserinus and posterior oblique fibers of the medial collateral ligament are left intact.

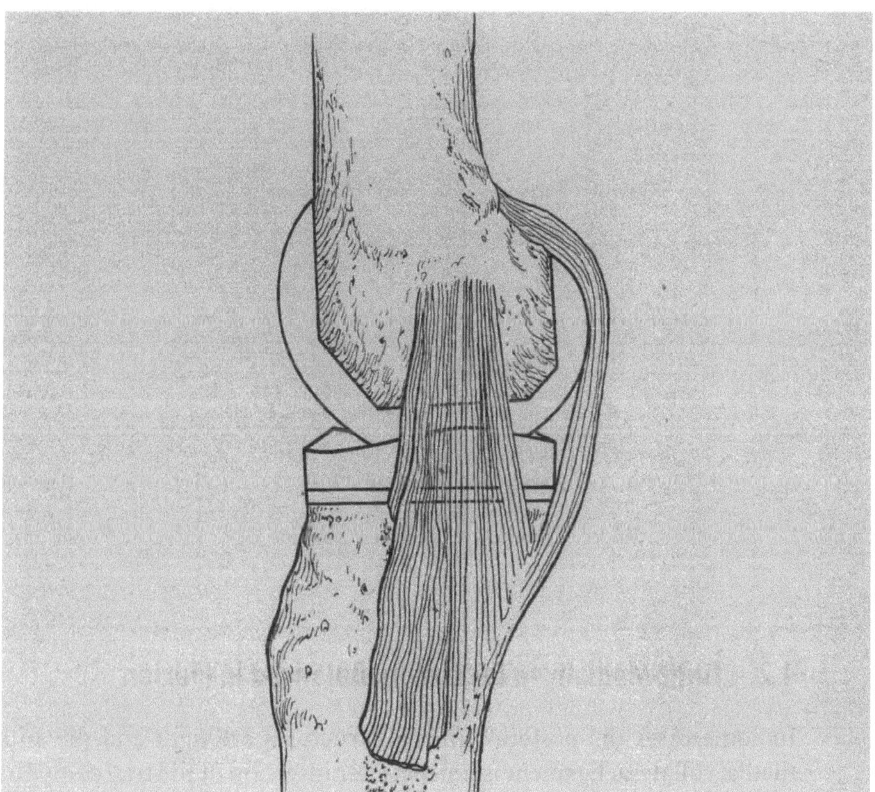

Fig. 71. The anterior fibers of the medial collateral ligament have been released. Medial stability in extension is near normal because the posterior portion of the medial collateral ligament and the posterior medial capsule function normally.

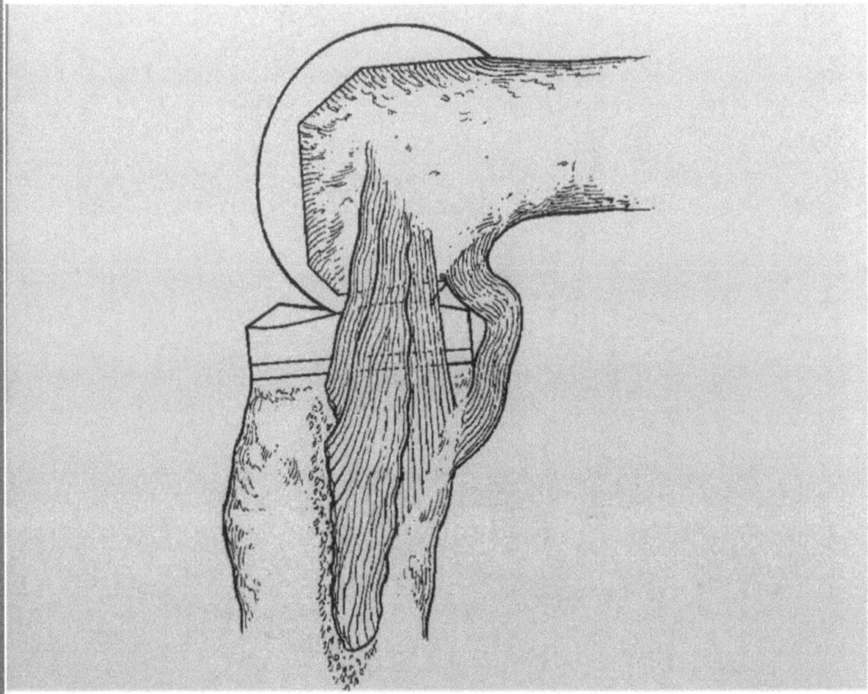

Fig. 72. In flexion the anterior medial collateral ligament is no longer tight. The posteromedial oblique portion of the medial collateral ligament now acts as a secondary medial stabilizer in flexion.

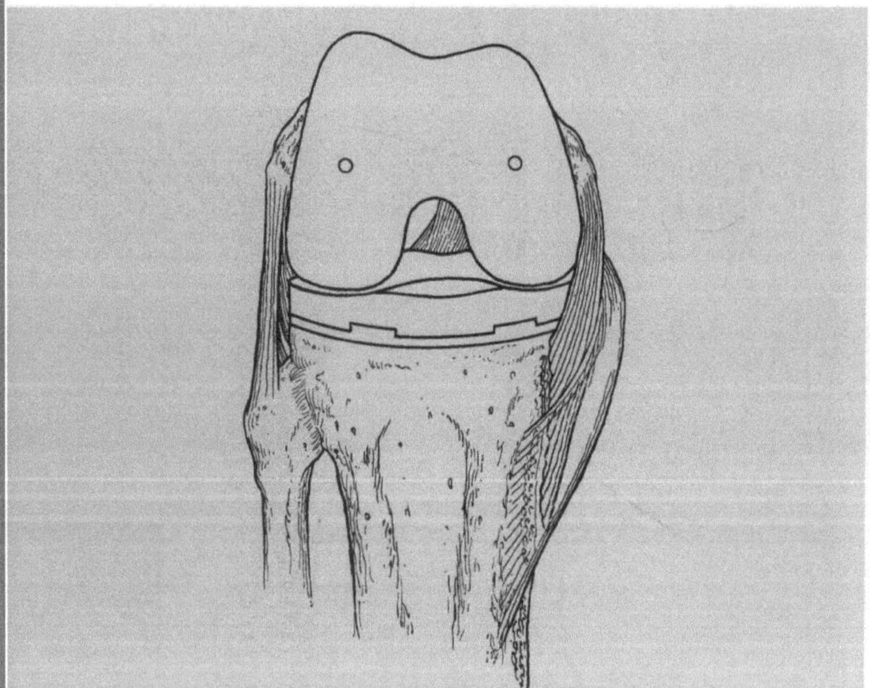

Fig. 73. On the anterior view, the medial femoral condyle sits in the center of the tibial surface, and the tibia pivots normally around the posterior cruciate ligament. The posterior cruciate ligament acts as a secondary varus-valgus stabilizer in flexion.

4.2. Tight Medially in Extension, Balanced in Flexion

In some cases the posterior medial structures are tight and the anterior medial collateral ligament is normal after insertion of the trial components. These knees are tight in extension, but balanced normally in flexion.

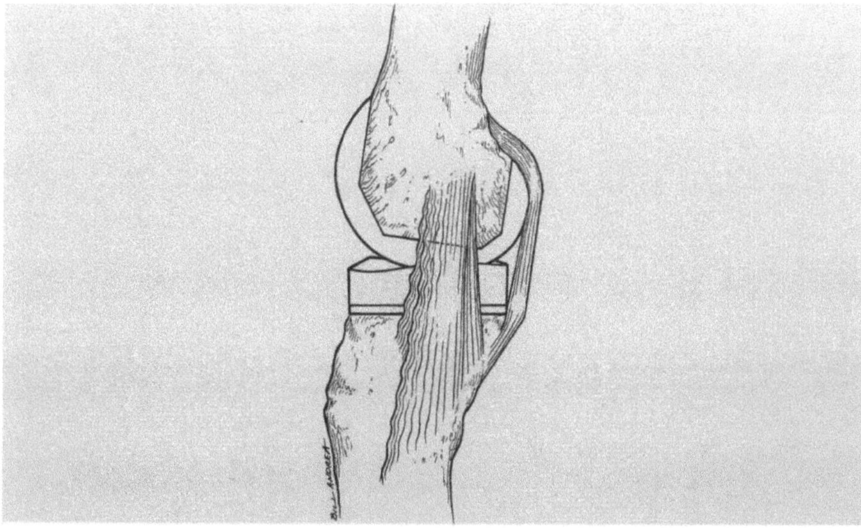

Fig. 74. In this case the knee does not extend quite fully. The posterior portion of the medial collateral ligament is tight and the posterior capsule also may be contracted. The anterior portion of the medial collateral ligament is loose in extension.

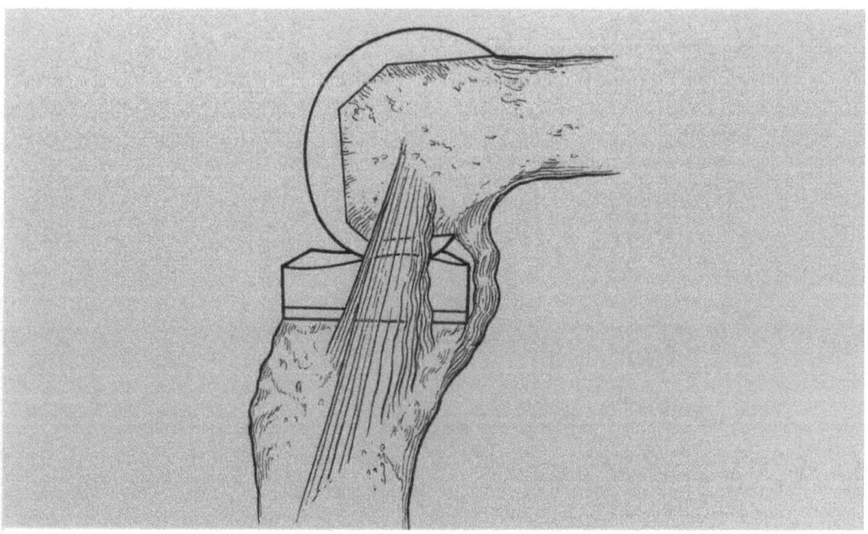

Fig. 75. In flexion the anterior medial collateral ligament fibers are brought to normal tension, and the posterior portion of the medial collateral ligament is slackened along with the medial posterior capsule. The knee has normal stability in flexion.

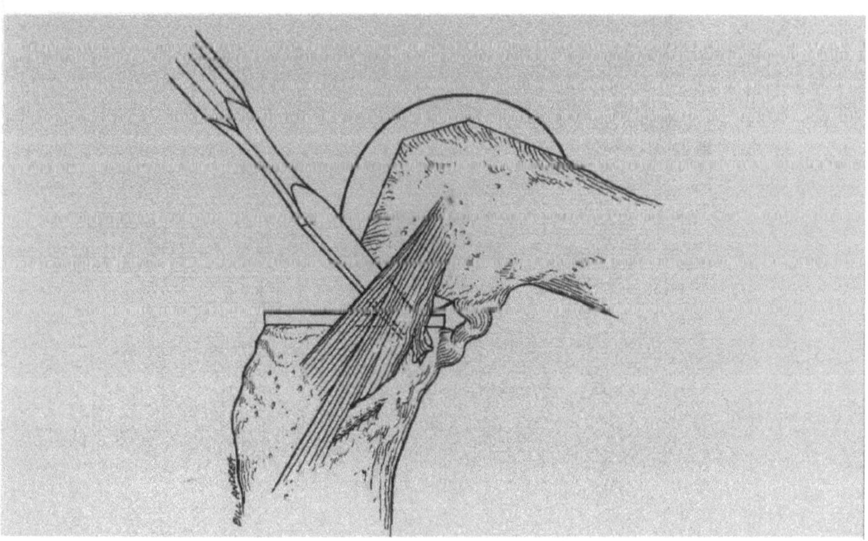

Fig. 76. In this case, only the posterior portion of the medial collateral ligament should be released first. A curved 1/2-inch osteotome is used to elevate all but the anterior portion of the medial collateral ligament. The osteotome is directed approximately 45° downward and tapped gently to release the postero-medial oblique fibers from the tibia and from the tendon of the semimembranosus.

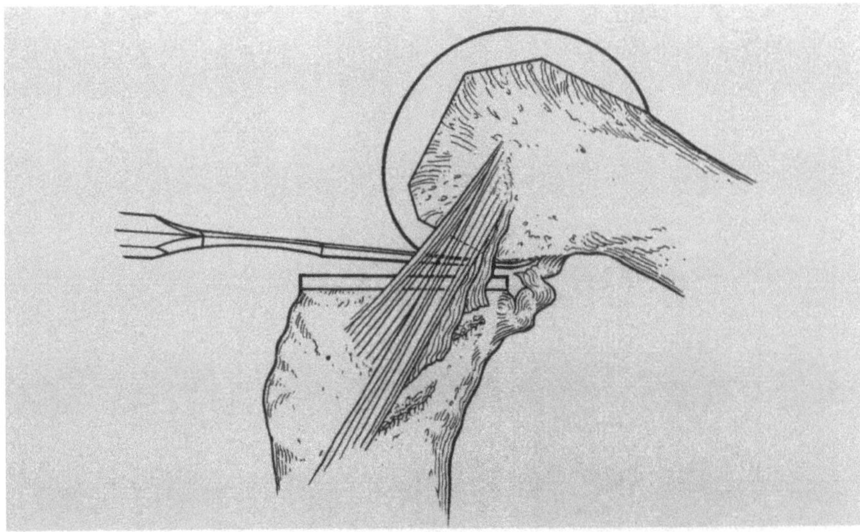

Fig. 77. If the knee still is too tight medially in extension but is well balanced in flexion, then the medial posterior capsule may be released. The curved 1/2-inch osteotome is used to gently elevate the capsule from the femur. Further posterior capsular release can be achieved by releasing the posterior capsule from the tibia as well (see flexion contracture section).

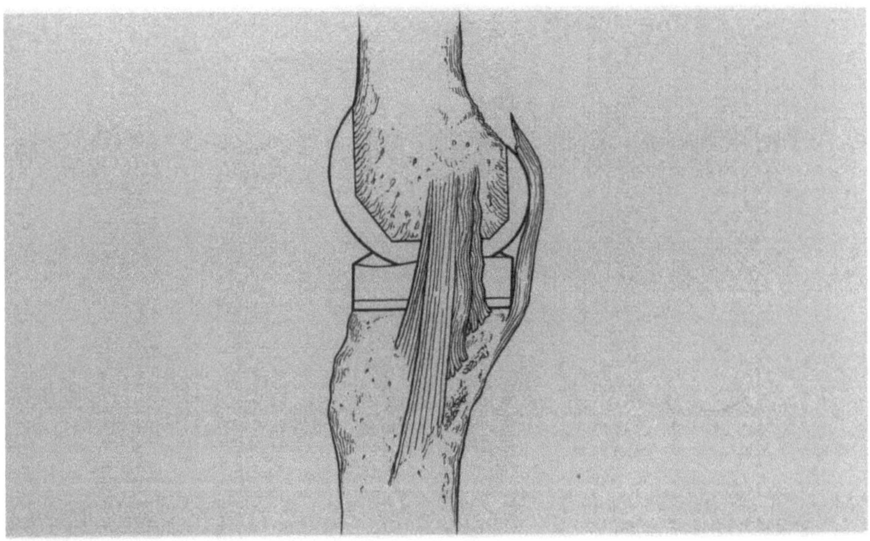

Fig. 78. The knee has had release of the medial posterior capsule and the posteromedial oblique fibers of the deep and superficial medial collateral ligament. The anterior fibers of the deep and superficial medial collateral ligament are still intact and afford medial stability in flexion and extension. The anterior edge of the medial collateral ligament, which normally is loose in extension, now has been brought into play, and acts as a secondary medial stabilizing structure.

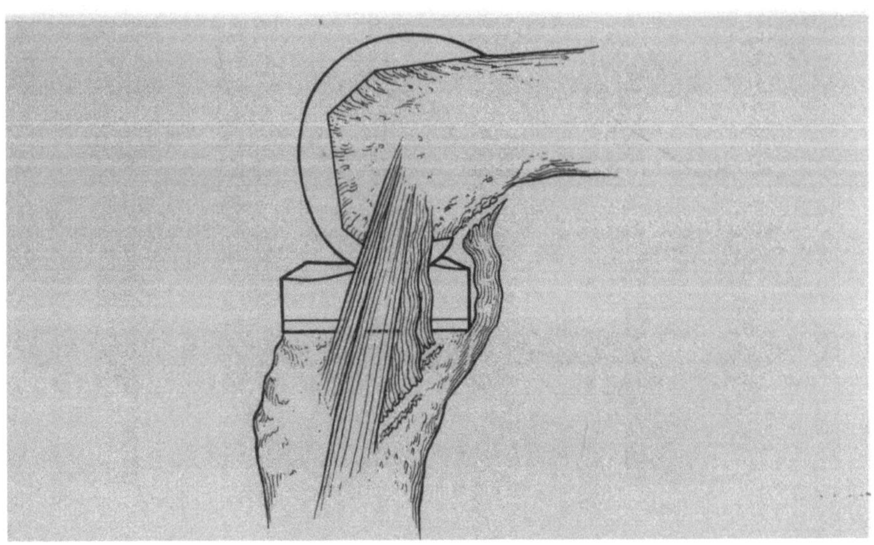

Fig. 79. With the knee flexed, the anterior portion of the medial collateral ligament tightens normally, providing normal medial stability to the knee.

4.3. Tight Medially in Flexion and Extension

In many cases with a long-standing varus deformity and medial ligament contracture, the knee is tight medially both in flexion and extension. This indicates that the entire medial collateral ligament is contracted. The posterior capsule and posterior cruciate ligament also may be contracted, but the primary contracture is the medial collateral ligament in these cases. The posterior cruciate ligament and posterior capsule cannot be evaluated until the medial collateral ligament contracture has been corrected.

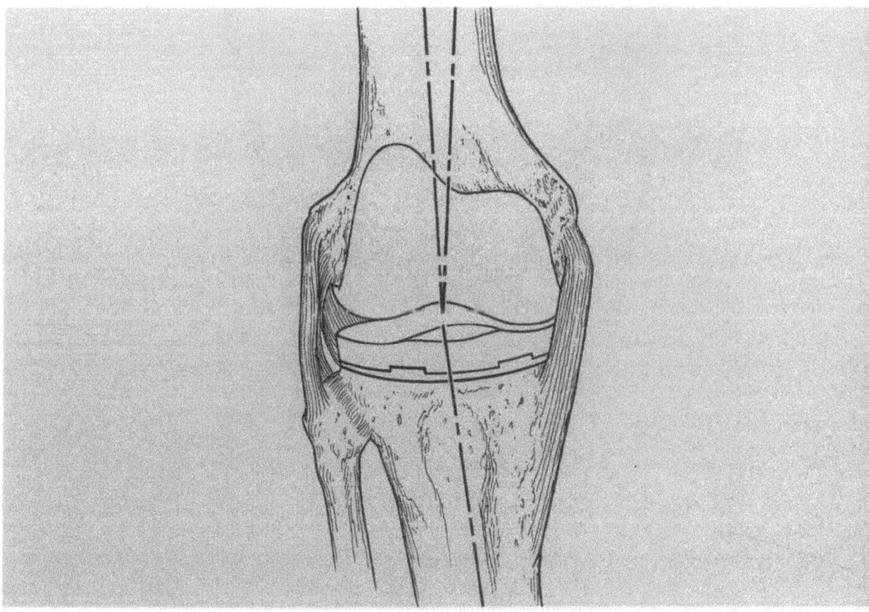

Fig. 80. In this illustration the knee is tight medially and gapes spontaneously laterally. It also has a 10° flexion contracture. The knee is still in varus malalignment due to ligament contracture despite correct alignment of the bone surface resection.

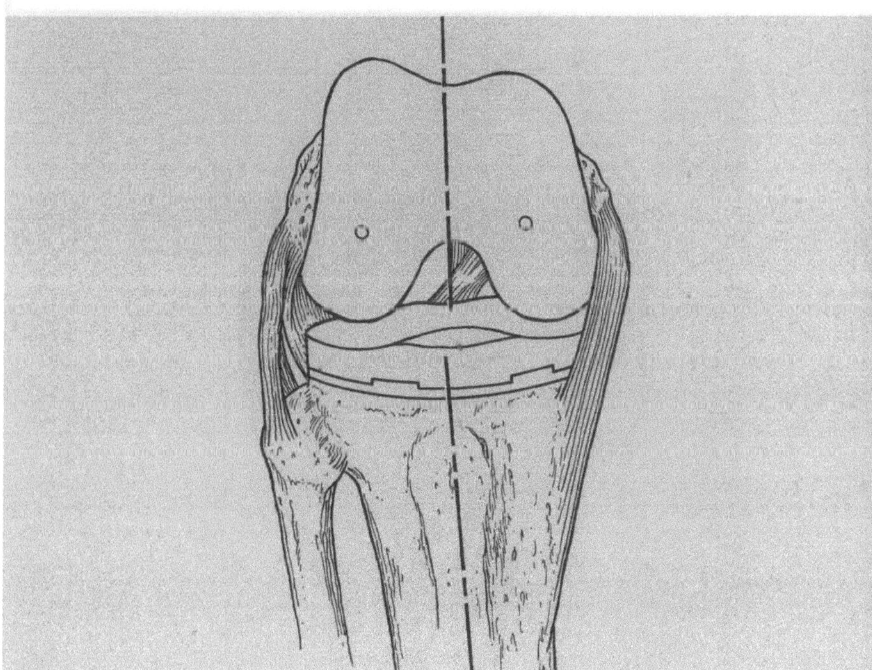

Fig. 81. The knee is tight medially in flexion as well. The knee is still in varus in flexion because of ligament imbalance despite correct alignment of the bone surface cuts. The lateral side gapes spontaneously, and the medial femoral condyle rolls to the posterior edge of the tibial spacer. The entire superficial medial collateral ligament, when palpated, feels tight in the flexed and extended positions. At this stage it is impossible to know if all medial structures including the posterior cruciate ligament and medial posterior capsule are tight, but it is clear that at least the anterior and posterior portions of the medial collateral ligament are tight.

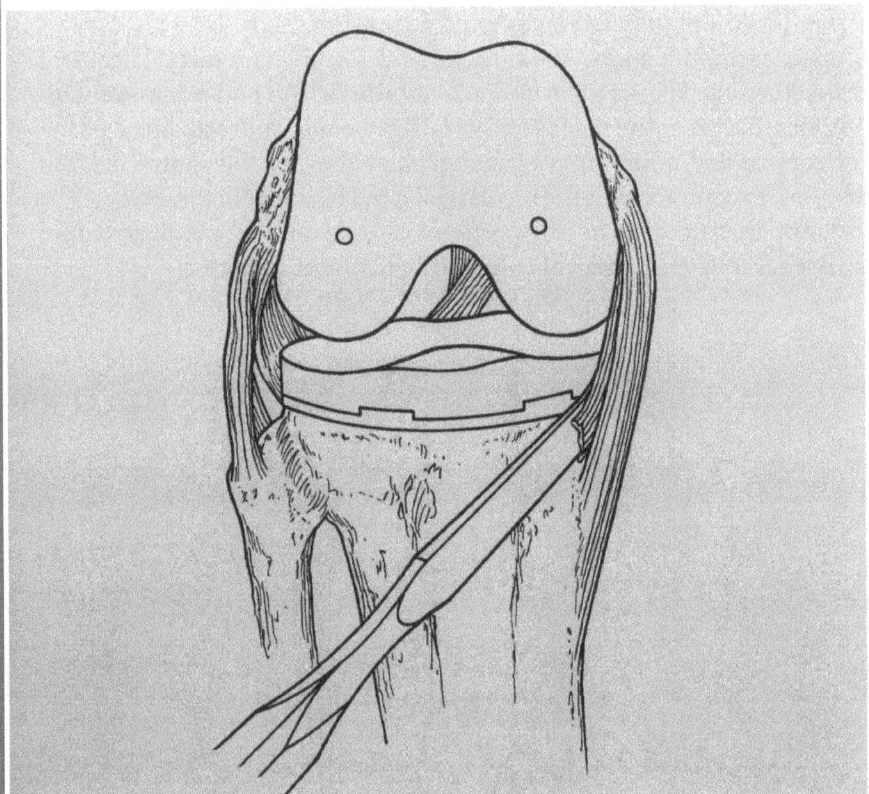

Fig. 82. Because the knee is tight medially both in flexion and extension, the entire medial collateral ligament is likely to be tight, but the posterior capsule and posterior cruciate ligament cannot yet be assessed. Because the anterior portion of the medial collateral ligament is more nearly isometric than the posterior, it is released first in hopes that it will be the only release necessary. The curved half-inch osteotome first is inserted at the upper, anterior edge of the medial collateral ligament.

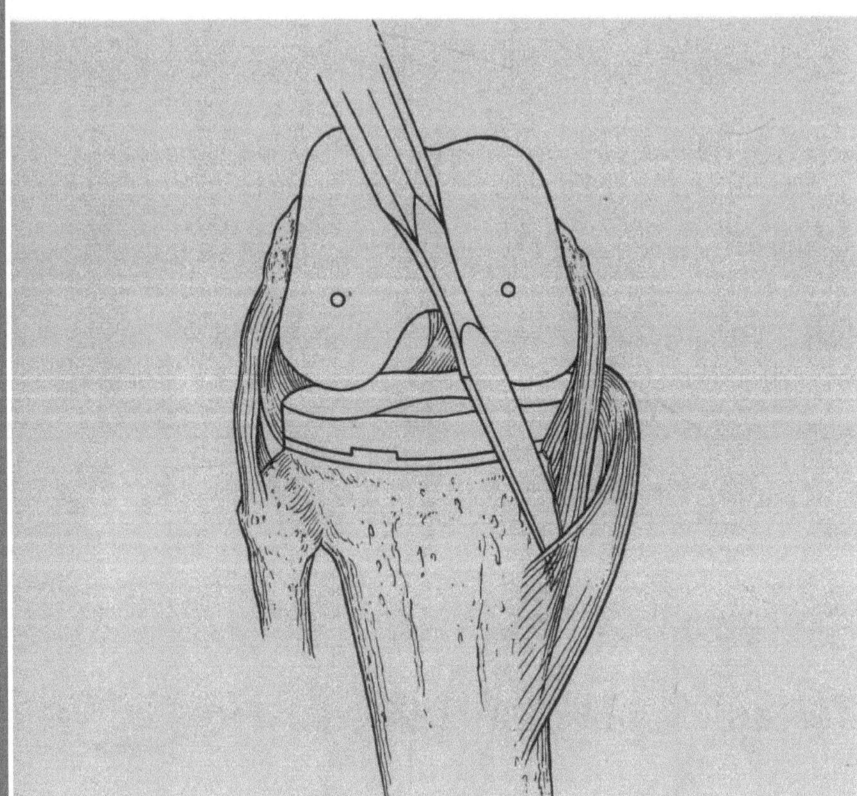

Fig. 83. The curved osteotome is placed beneath the superficial medial collateral ligament just behind the insertion of the pes anserinus, and the anterior portion of the deep and superficial medial collateral ligament is stripped subperiosteally from the tibia first. Because the anterior fibers have some effect both in flexion and extension, this often is sufficient. However, in most cases it is necessary to strip the posterior portion from its attachments as well.

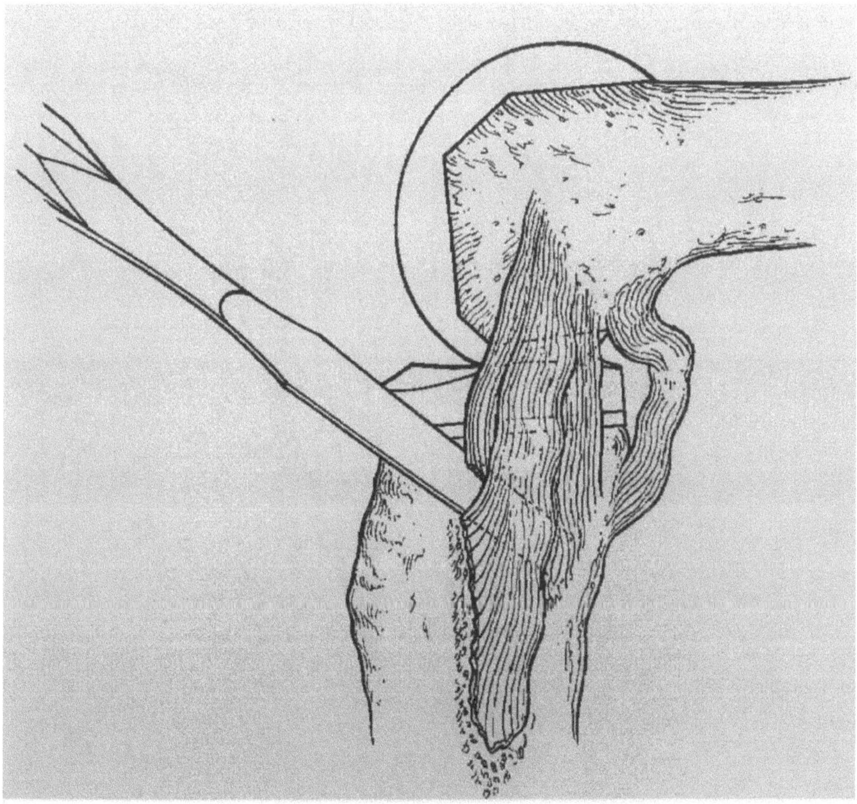

Fig. 84. If the knee remains tight medially in extension after release of the anterior medial collateral ligament fibers, then the posterior fibers are released. Here the curved half-inch osteotome is passed under the released anterior fibers and angled downward 45° to release the posterior oblique fibers of the medial collateral ligament. The medial collateral ligament maintains loose attachment to the pes anserinus, and the distal periosteal attachments to the ligament remain intact as well, so the knee does not become grossly lax as a result of this procedure. The secondary medial stabilizers (the medial posterior capsule in extension and the posterior cruciate ligament in flexion) also are called into play, and prevent destabilization of the knee.

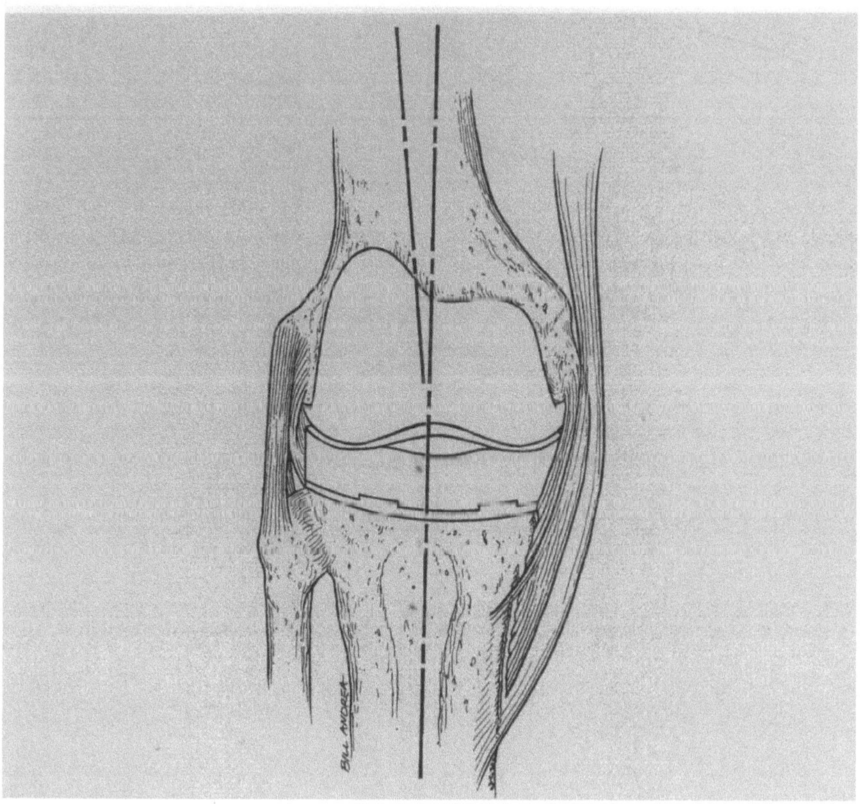

Fig. 85. A thicker tibial component has been added to tension all ligaments. The deep and superficial medial collateral ligaments are free of their distal attachments to bone, but remain attached to the periosteum and deep fascia. Now the knee extends fully. The stretched lateral structures are brought to normal tension by the additional tibial thickness. The varus deformity has been corrected, and the mechanical axis of the femur is aligned with the long axis of the tibia.

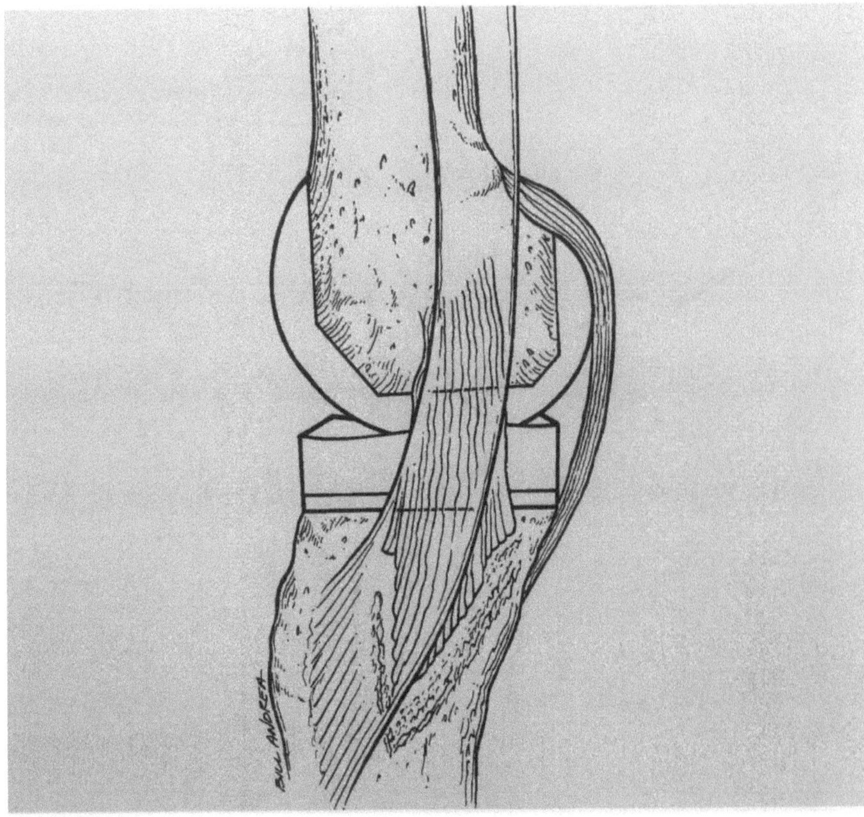

Fig. 86. The flexion contracture has been corrected by releasing the medial collateral ligament. Now the posterior capsule is brought to appropriate tension as the knee extends fully, and acts as a secondary medial stabilizer in extension. If the knee will not extend fully, the medial posterior capsule is the only remaining tight structure, and may be released using the technique illustrated in Figures 77, 78, 174 and 175.

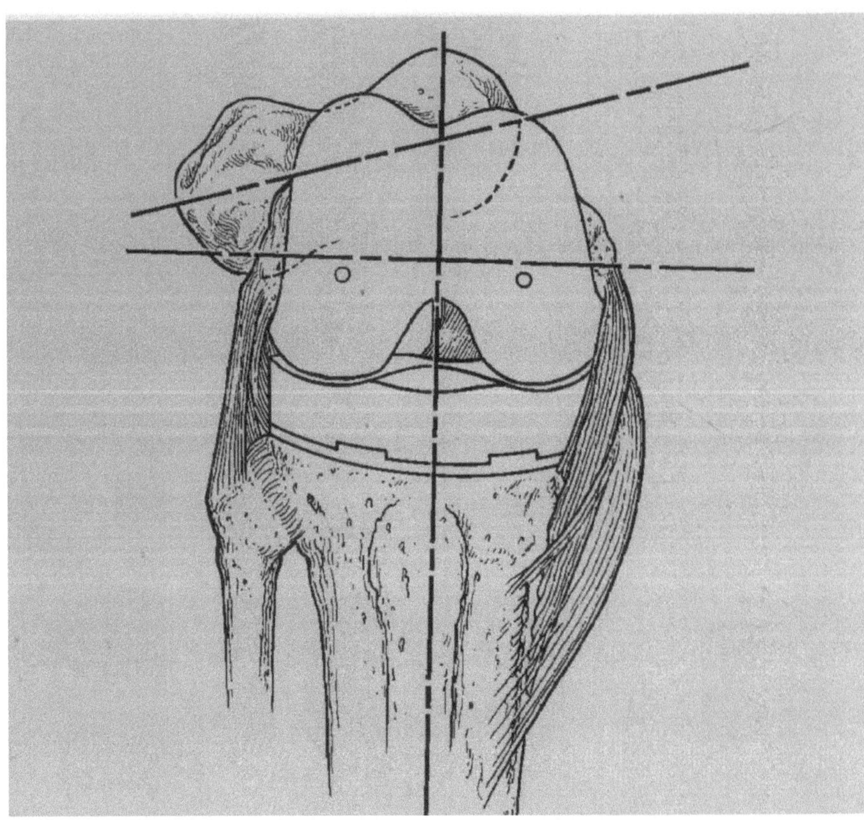

Fig. 87. The effect is similar in flexion. Now the femoral surface is seated correctly on the medial tibial surface. The posterior cruciate ligament functions as a secondary varus-valgus stabilizer in flexion. The anterior-posterior axis of the femur passes through the center of the femoral head and aligns correctly with the long axis of the tibia.

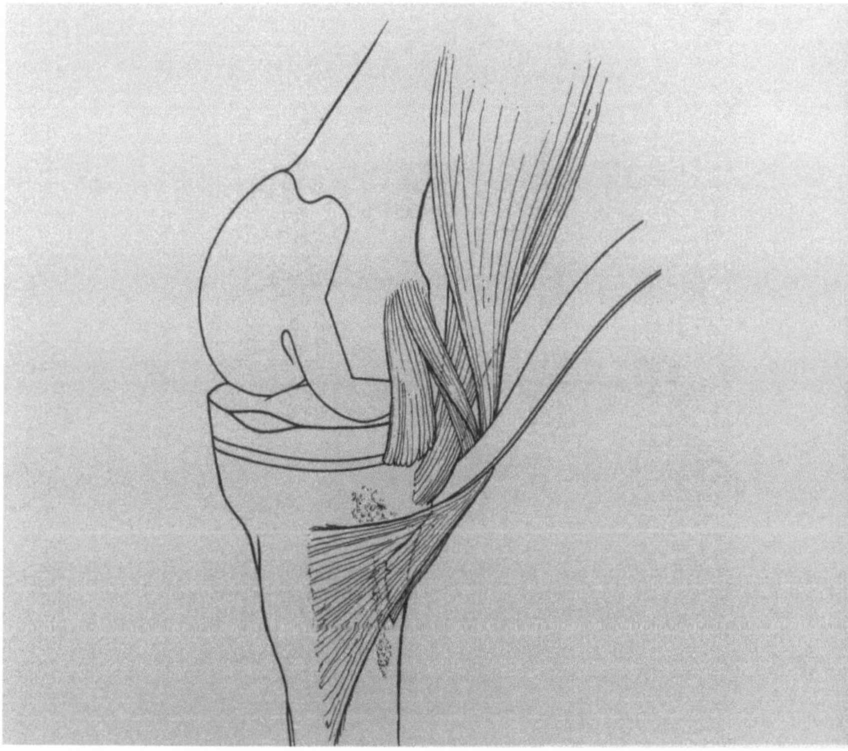

Fig. 88. Rarely, after release of the medial collateral ligament, the knee is still unacceptably tight medially because of contracted semimembranosus and pes anserinus. These structures should be released from the tibia in these rare circumstances. The semimembranosus attachment can be exposed by placing a Hohman retractor behind the posterior medial edge of the tibial flare. The pes anserinus attachment is accessible by extending the subperiosteal release of the medial collateral ligament anteriorly to include the tendon fibers.

4.4. Tight Popliteus Tendon

Occasionally the popliteus tendon and its surrounding structures are tight in the varus knee after the medial side has been corrected. This often is difficult to detect, but rotational stability testing of the tibia demonstrates that the tibia is held anteriorly on the lateral side and pivots around the lateral edge of the tibial component.

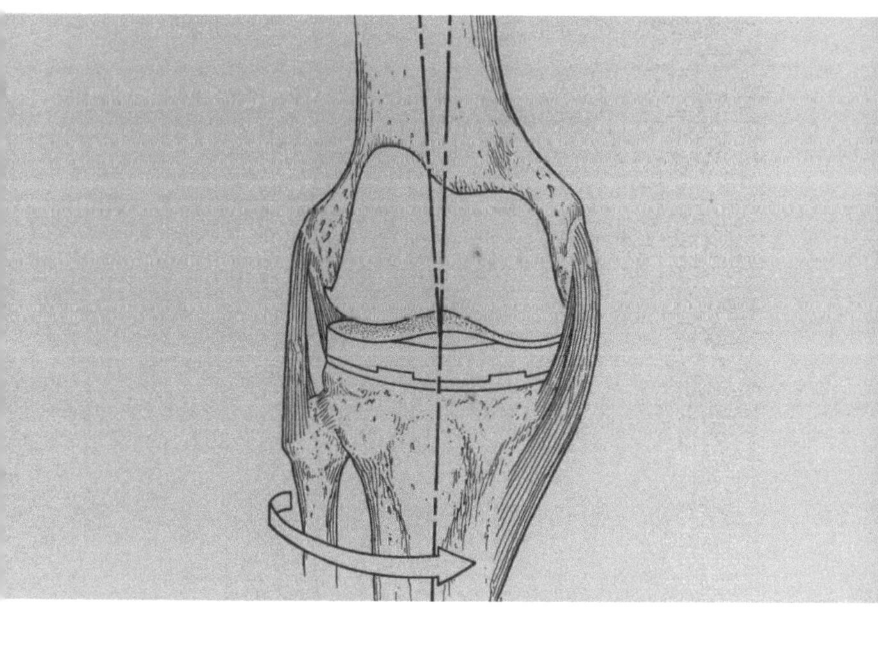

Fig. 89. The tibia is held internally rotated by the tight popliteus tendon, and the femoral surface seats far posteriorly on the tibial surface.

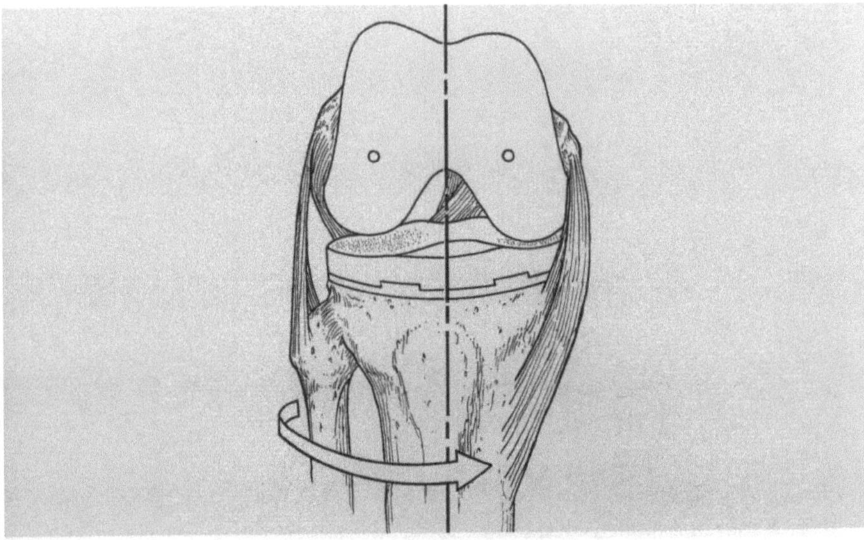

Fig. 90. In the flexed position the internal rotational malposition of the tibia is more apparent. The tibia pivots around the tight popliteus tendon. When the tibia is rotated around its long axis, very little movement occurs laterally, and near normal movement occurs medially.

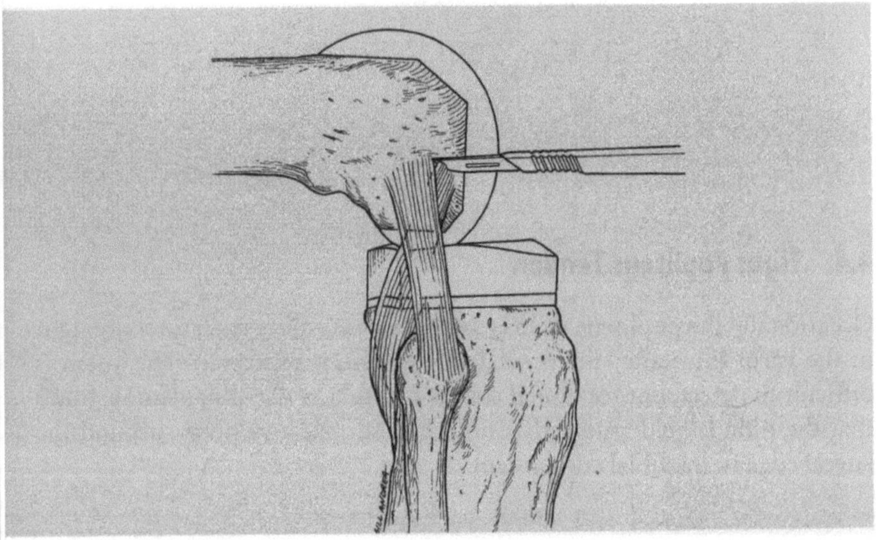

Fig. 91. The lateral tibial surface is held abnormally far anteriorly by the tight popliteus complex. The popliteus tendon is released from its bone attachment with the knee flexed. It is found just distal and posterior to the lateral collateral ligament attachment, and care must be taken to avoid release of the lateral collateral ligament during this procedure.

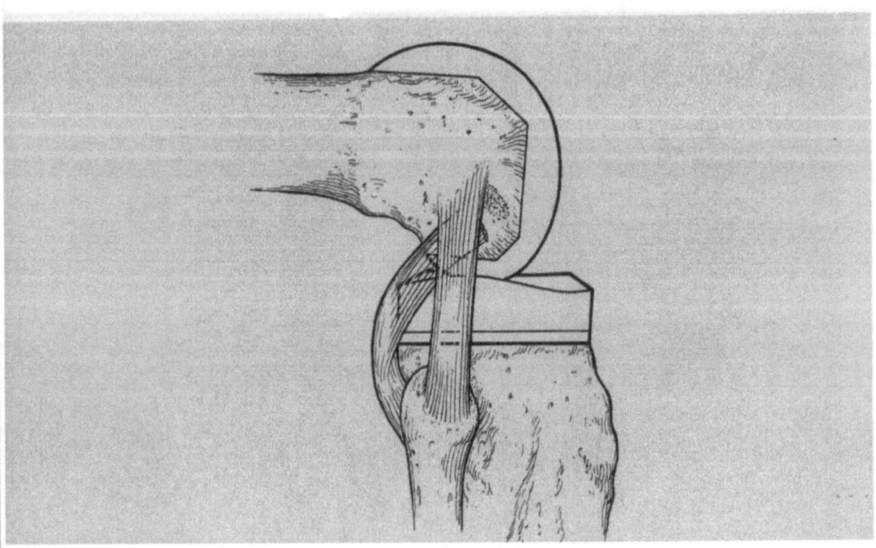

Fig. 92. The popliteus tendon has been released from its attach-ment to the femur and has slid posteriorly, allowing the tibia to move posteriorly as well. Now the femur sits normally on the tibial surface.

4.5. Compensatory Lateral Release -Extension only

Occasionally, after full medial collateral ligament release, the knee is excessively loose on the medial side in extension, and tight laterally. Compensatory lateral release corrects the imbalance, and a thicker tibial component brings the knee to correct stability.

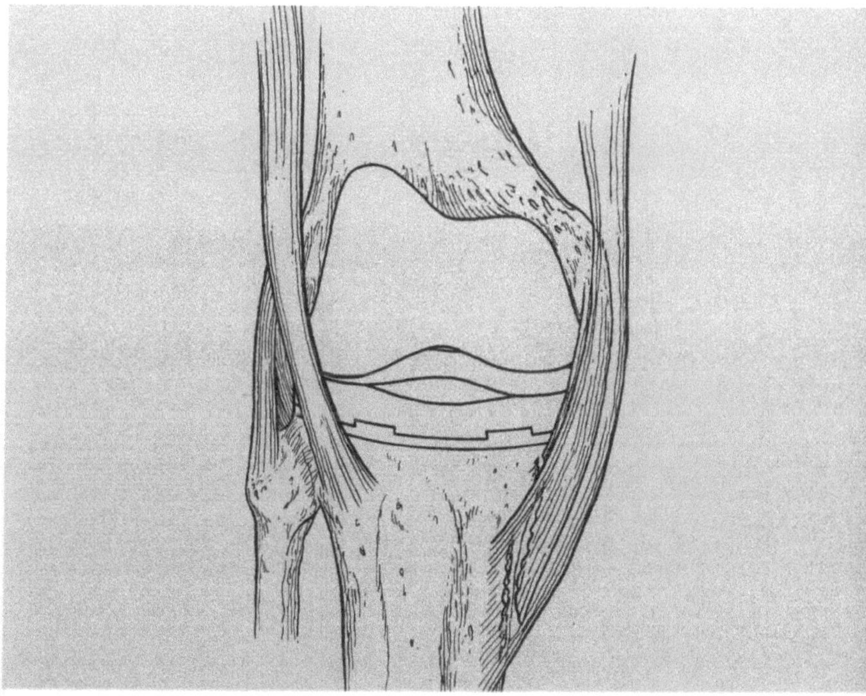

Fig. 93. After medial collateral ligament release, the knee gapes medially and is tight laterally in extension.

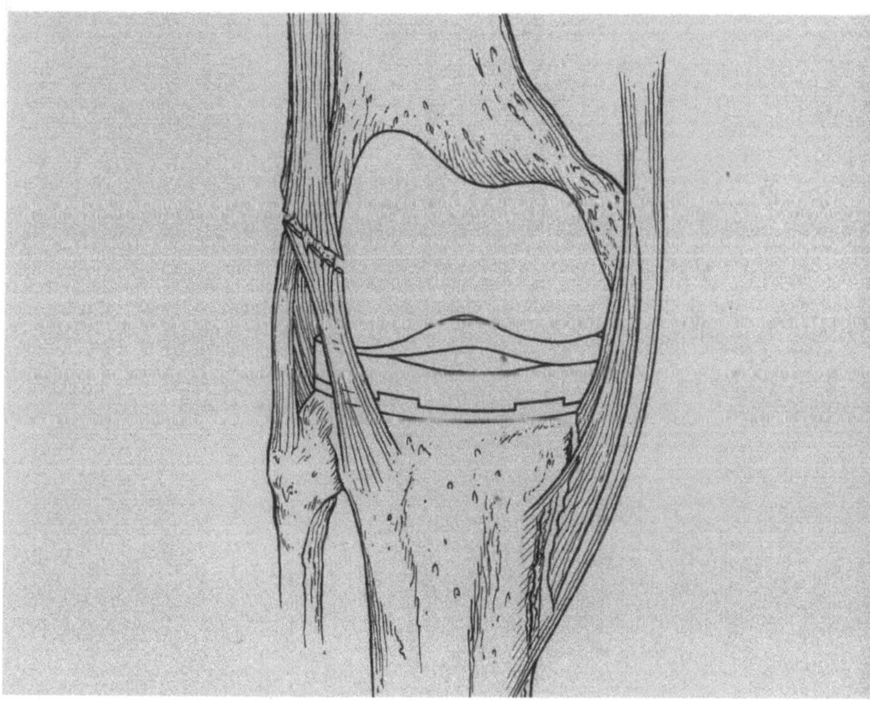

Fig. 94. To correct this imbalance, the iliotibial band is released to create more space in extension

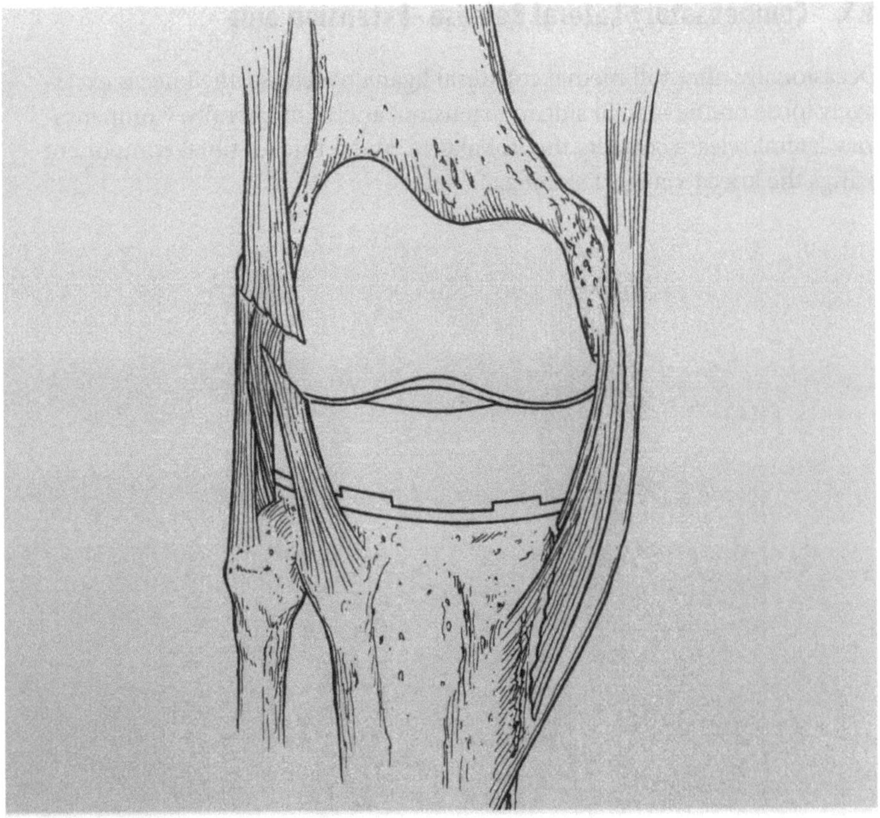

Fig. 95. A thicker tibial component is added, bringing the knee to correct medial-lateral ligament balance in extension. The lateral collateral ligament and popliteus tendon are tensioned on the lateral side, and the periosteal attachments of the medial collateral ligament are placed under tension.

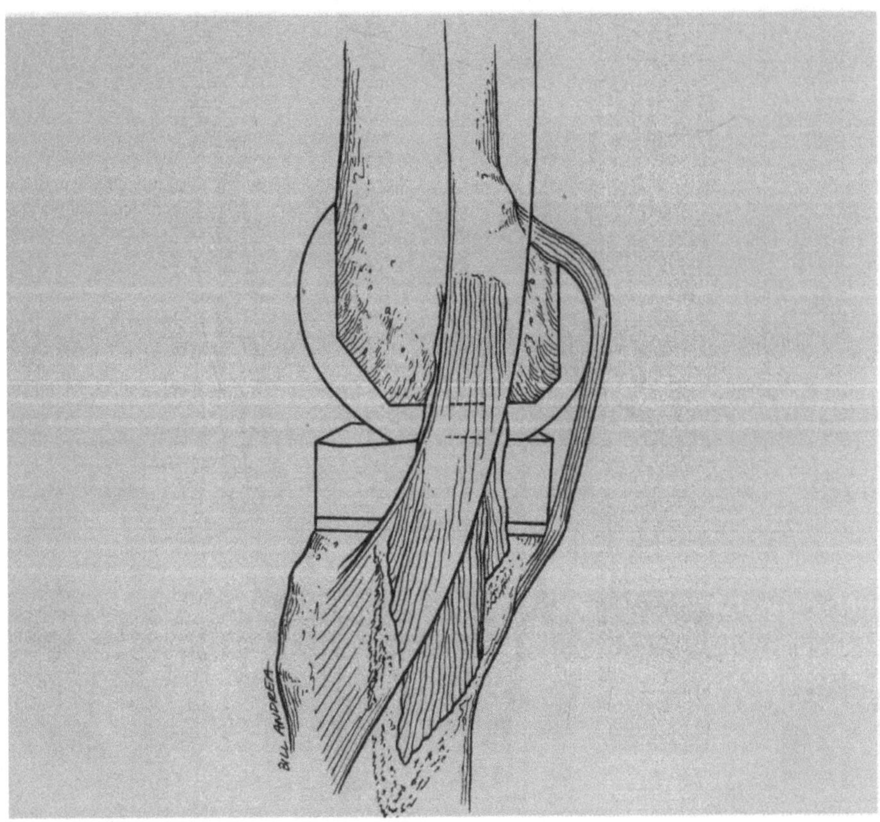

Fig. 96. Also, the medial posterior capsule, an important secondary medial stabilizer, is brought to tension to enhance this secondary role.

4.6. Compensatory Lateral Release – Flexion and Extension

In some cases after full release of the medial collateral ligament, the secondary stabilizers are inadequate to provide medial stability in flexion and extension, and the knee is too loose medially after the tibial component has been sized to bring the lateral ligaments to their normal tension. In those cases the lateral collateral ligament and popliteus tendon are released to create more laxity both in flexion and extension, and a thicker tibial component is used to tension the medial structures.

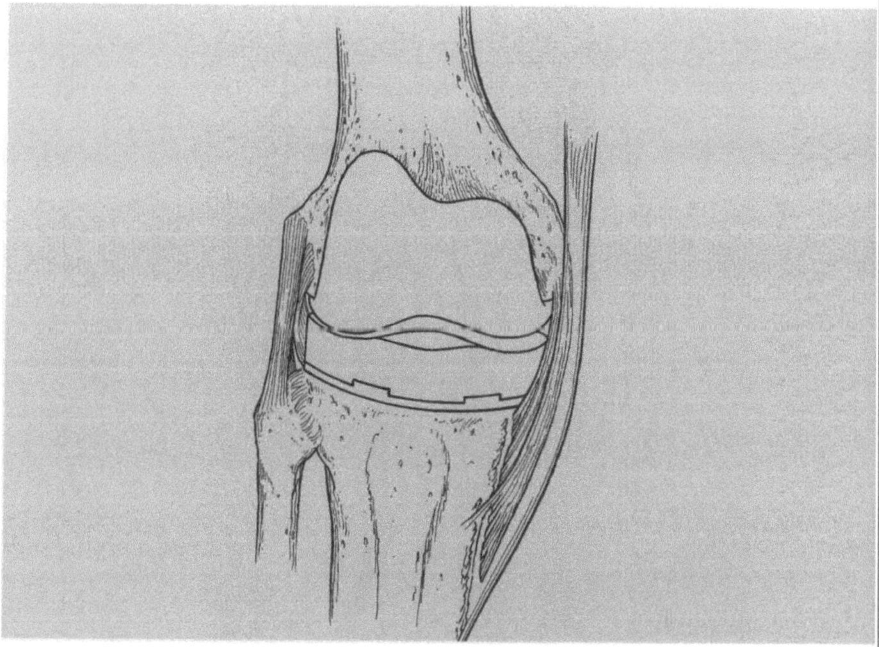

Fig. 97. The knee is loose medially in extension after medial collateral ligament release.

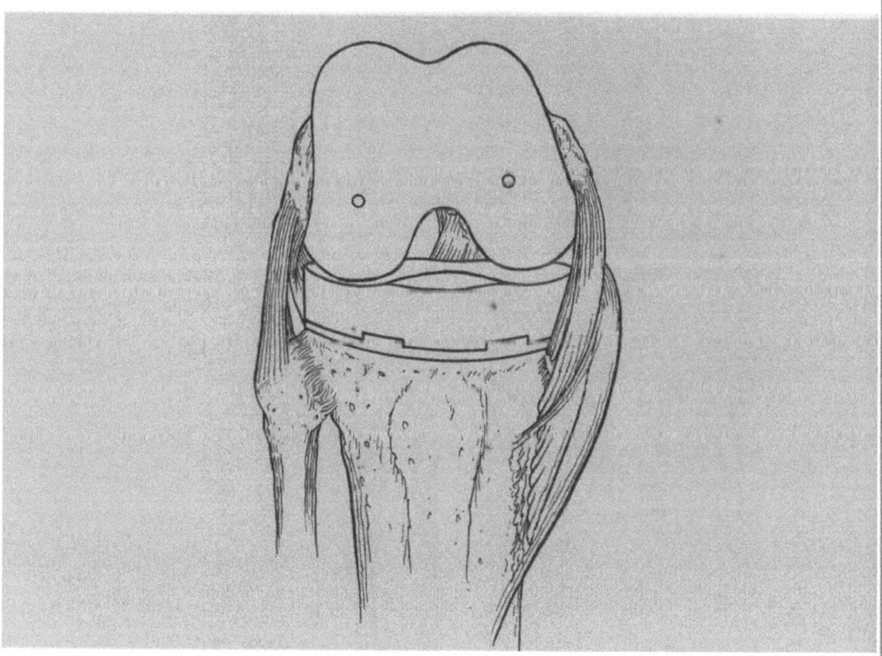

Fig. 98. The medial side also is loose in flexion.

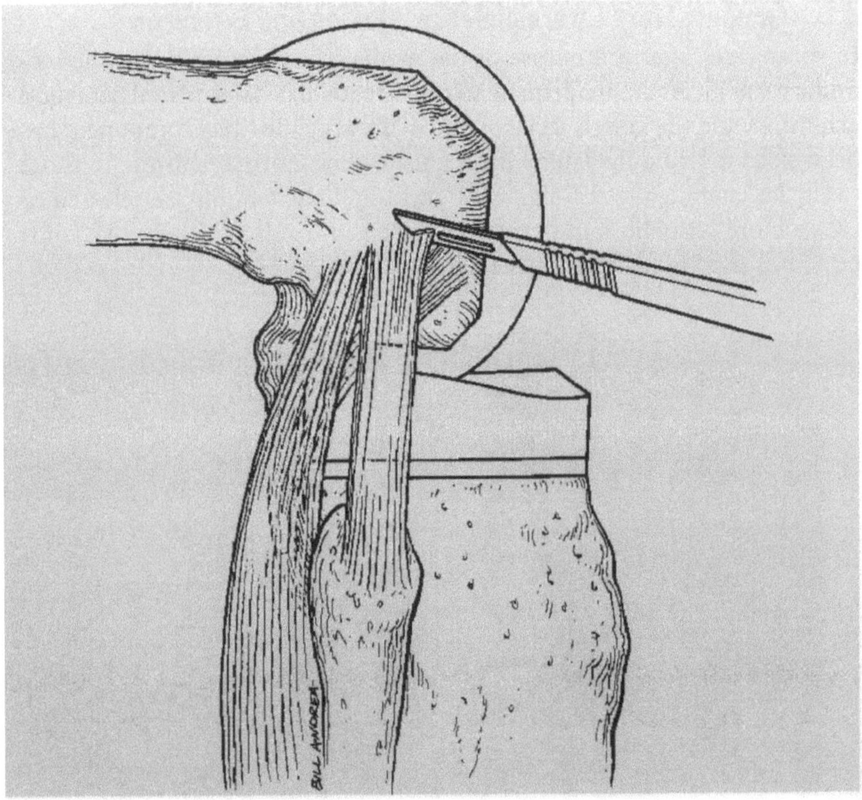

Fig. 99. Compensatory release of the lateral collateral ligament makes room for a larger tibial spacer especially in extension, but has some effect through the entire flexion arc. This release is done with a knife, releasing the lateral collateral ligament directly from the bone, but leaving it attached to the surrounding dense fibrous capsule, and to the popliteus tendon. Compensatory release of the popliteus tendon is done if more laxity is needed primarily in flexion. The lateral posterior capsule and posterolateral corner act as secondary stabilizing structures if releases of the lateral collateral ligament and popliteus tendon are necessary.

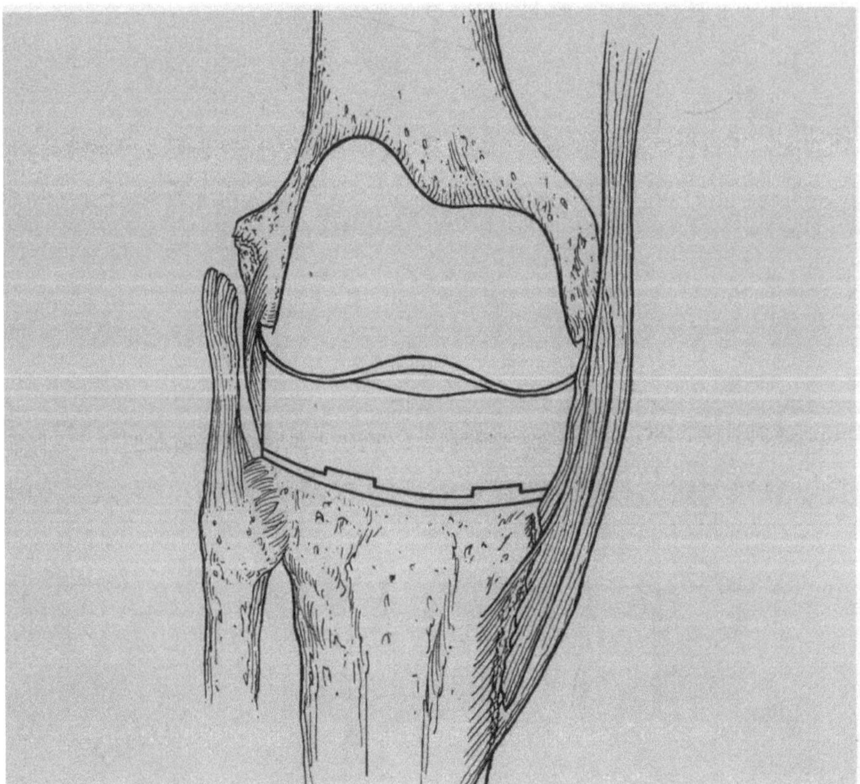

Fig. 100. A thicker polyethylene spacer tensions the knee appro-priately, tensioning the iliotibial band and posterior capsule in extension. In some cases the iliotibial band must be partially released to create a little more compensatory lateral relaxation in the extended position.

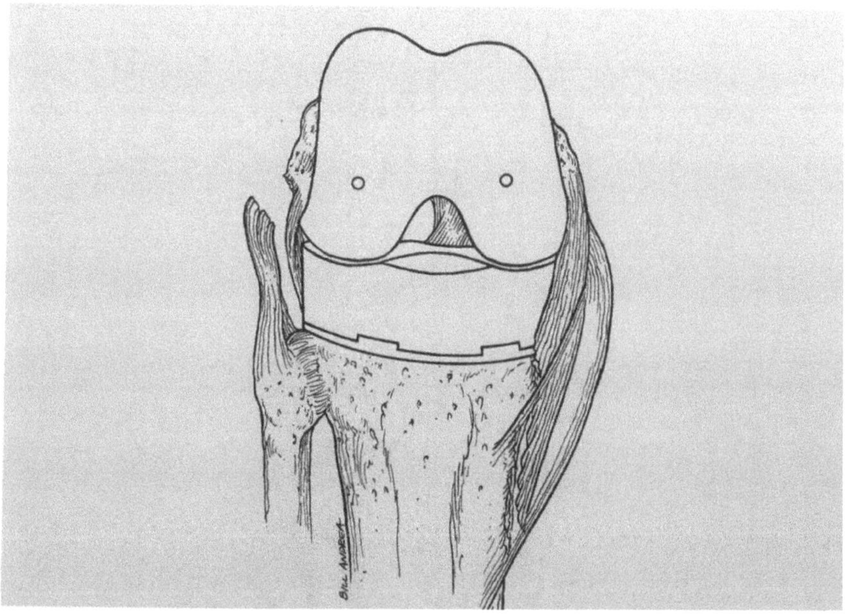

Fig. 101. In flexion the posterior cruciate ligament acts as the major secondary stabilizer. Also, the popliteus tendon or lateral collateral ligament, if not released, will act as a secondary lateral stabilizing structure.

4.7. Pitfalls of the Varus Knee

One of the most common causes of instability and patellar tracking problems in the varus knee is the practice of early release of the medial collateral ligament in extension, and then using tensioners to balance the flexion space.

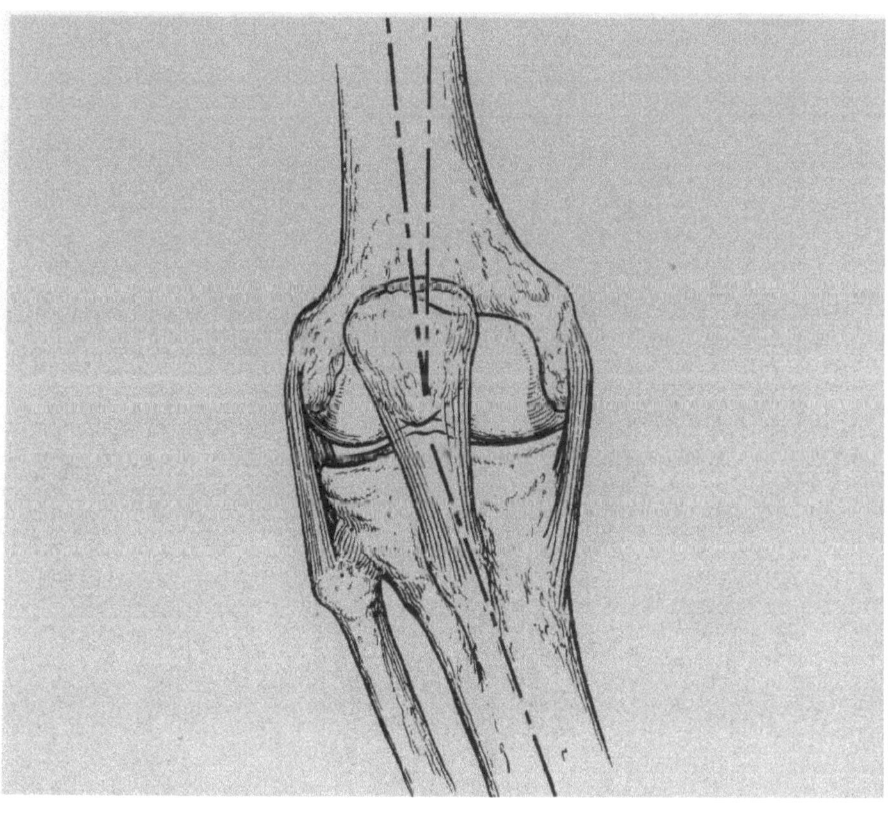

Fig. 102. The varus knee has medial tibial collapse and contracture of the medial collateral ligament.

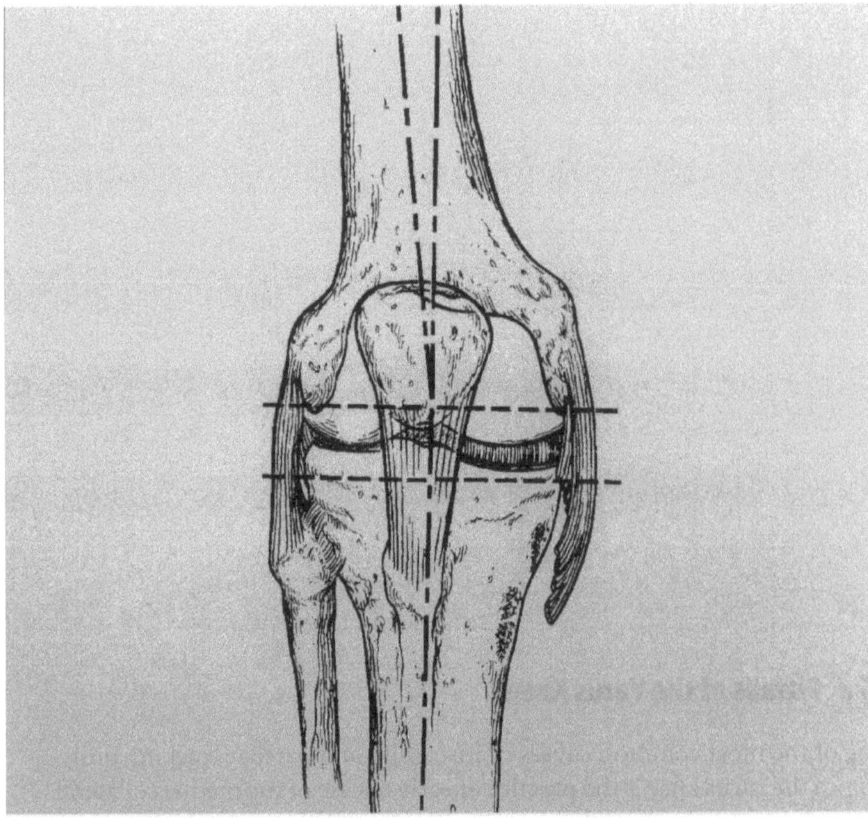

Fig. 103. Full release of the medial collateral ligament allows correction of the deformity in extension. The posterior capsule is the secondary medial stabilizer, and maintains normal medial stability in extension.

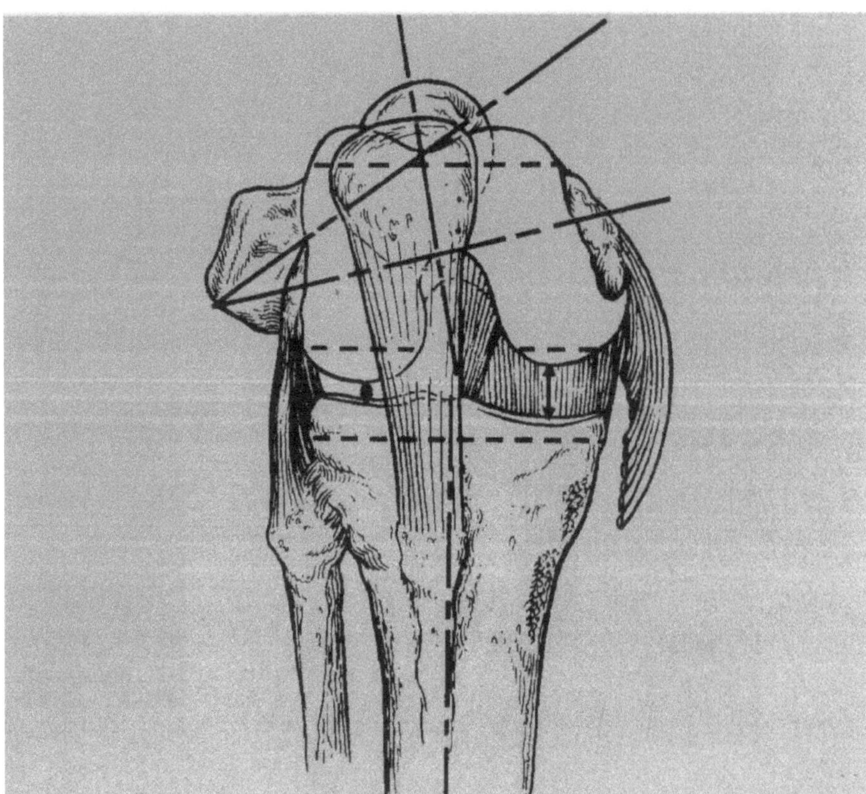

Fig. 104. In flexion, when the tensioners are applied, the medial joint is distracted until the posterior cruciate ligament or the medial posterior capsule, which normally are not tight in flexion, actually are tightened. This externally rotates the femur and the hip joint, tilts the epicondylar axis laterally, and positions the patellar groove laterally. The tibia is now angled toward valgus relative to the femur in flexion. The bone surface cuts are made parallel to the tibial surface. The knee will be stable, but alignment will be in excessive valgus in flexion, and the new position of the patellar groove will be medialized.

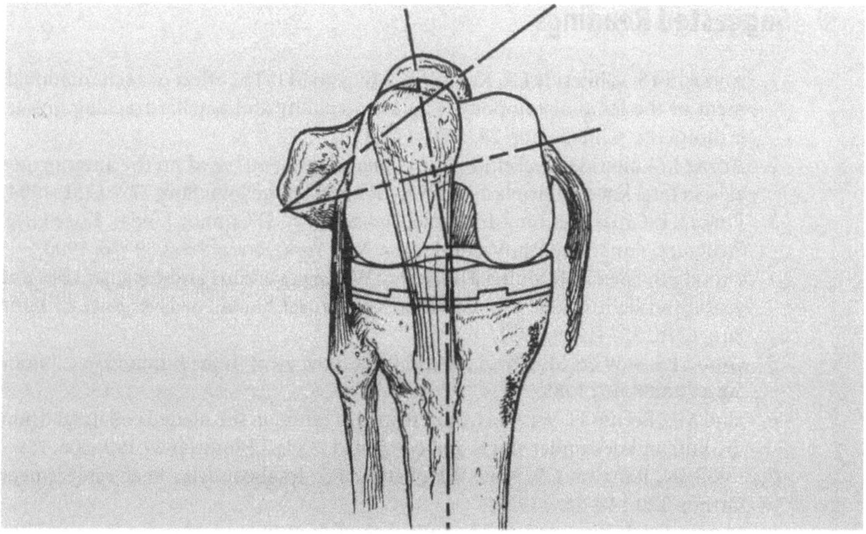

Fig. 105. The components have been inserted. The femur and hip are still externally rotated. The epicondylar axis is tilted laterally, and the patella is still positioned laterally. The new patellar groove is positioned medially relative to the femoral head, epicondylar axis, and patella.

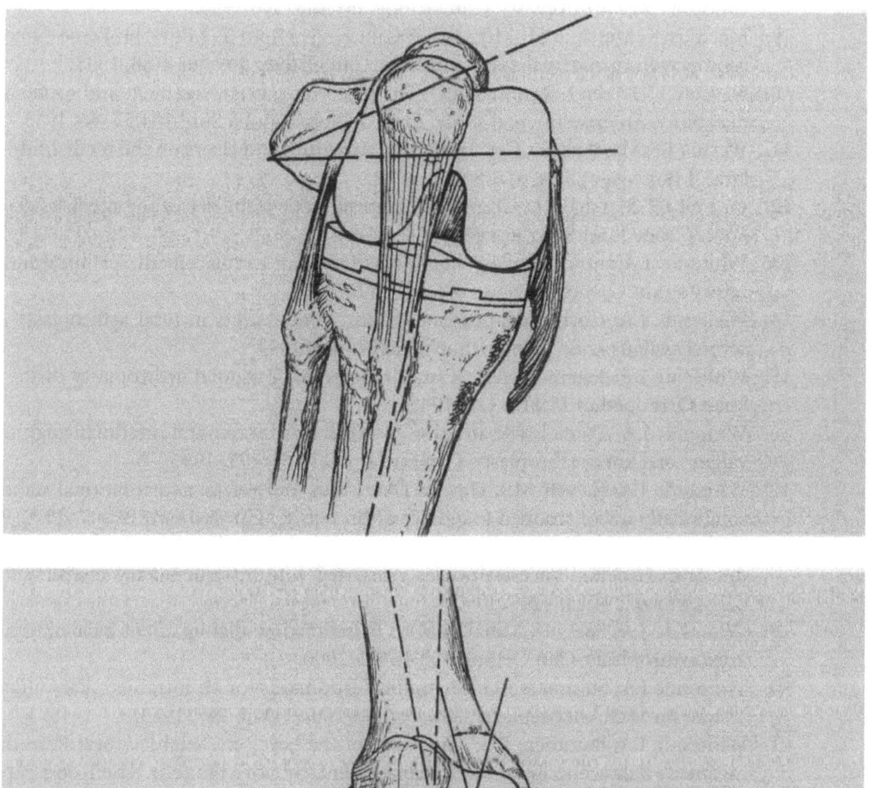

Fig. 106. When the hip is allowed to return to its normal functional position, the epicondylar axis is parallel with the ground, and the tibia is aligned in valgus. The long axis of the tibia passes through this new patellar groove, but not through the center of the femoral head. The patella is positioned laterally.

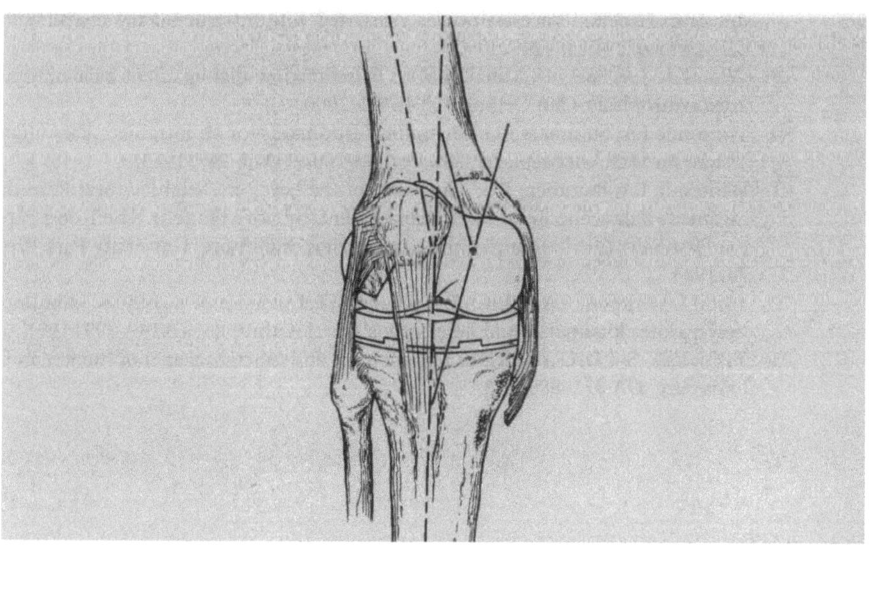

Fig. 107. When the knee is extended, it is stable, and varus-valgus alignment is correct. However, the femoral component is internally rotated, and the patellar groove is medialized. The patella still sits lateral to the new patellar groove. When the patella is placed in the patellar groove, the Q-angle is excessive, approximately 30° in this illustration.

Suggested Readings

1. Anouchi YS, Whiteside LA, Kaiser AD, Milliano MT: The effect of axial rotational alignment of the femoral component on knee stability and patellar tracking in total knee arthroplasty. Clin Orthop 287:170–177, 1991.
2. Arima J, Whiteside LA: Femoral rotational alignment, based on the anterior-posterior axis, in total knee arthroplasty in a valgus knee. J Bone Joint Surg 77A:1331–1334, 1995.
3. Burks RT: Gross Anatomy. In Daniel D, Akeson W, O'Connor J (eds). Knee Ligaments: Structure, Function, Injury, and Repair. New York, Raven Press 59–76, 1990.
4. Grood ES, Noyes FR, Butler DJ, Suntay WJ: Ligamentous and capsular restraints preventing straight medial and lateral laxity in intact human cadaver knees. J Bone Joint Surg 63A:1257–1269, 1981.
5. Grood ES, Stowers SF, Noyes FR: Limits of movement in the human knee. J Bone Joint Surg 70A:88–97, 1988.
6. Hull ML, Berns GS, Varma H, Patterson HA: Strain in the medial collateral ligament of the human knee under single and combined loads. J Biomech 29:199–206, 1996.
7. Insall JN, Ranawat CS, Scott WN, Walker PS: Total condylar knee replacement. Clin Orthop 120:149–154, 1976.
8. Martin JW, Whiteside LA: The influence of joint line position on knee stability after condylar knee arthroplasty. Clin Orthop 259:146–156,1990.
9. Matsuda S, Matsuda H, Miyagi T, Sasaki K, Iwamoto Y, Miura H: Femoral condyle geometry in the normal and varus knee. Clin Orthop 349:183–188, 1998.
10. Nielson S, Ovesen J, Rasmussen O: The posterior cruciate ligament and rotatory knee instability. An experimental study. Arch Orthop Trauma Surg 104:53–56, 1985.
11. Warren LF, Marshall JL: The supporting structures and layers on the medial side of the knee. J Bone Joint Surg 61A:56–62, 1979.
12. Warren LF, Marshall JL, Girgis F: The prime static stabilizer of the medial side of the knee. J Bone Joint Surg 56A:665–674, 1974.
13. Whiteside LA: Intramedullary alignment of total knee replacement. A clinical and laboratory study. Orthop Review (suppl) 9–12, 1989.
14. Whiteside LA: Correction of ligament and bone defects in total arthroplasty of the severely valgus knee. Clin Orthop 288:234–245, 1993.
15. Whiteside LA: Ligament release and bone grafting in total arthroplasty of the varus knee. Orthopedics 18:117–122, 1995.
16. Whiteside LA, Arima J: The anterior-posterior axis for femoral rotational alignment in valgus total knee arthroplasty. Clin Orthop 321:168–172, 1995.
17. Whiteside LA, Kasselt MR, Haynes DW: Varus and valgus and rotational stability in rotationally unconstrained total knee arthroplasty. Clin Orthop 219:147–157, 1987.
18. Whiteside LA, McCarthy DS: Laboratory evaluation of alignment and kinematics in a unicompartmental knee arthroplasty inserted with intramedullary instrumentation. Clin Orthop 274:238–247, 1992.
19. Whiteside LA, Saeki K, Mihalko MW: Functional medial ligament balancing in total knee arthroplasty. Clin Orthop 380:45–57, 2000.
20. Whiteside LA, Summers RG: Anatomical landmarks for an intramedullary alignment system for total knee replacement. Orthop Trans 7:546–547, 1983.
21. Whiteside LA, Summers RG: The Effect of the Level of Distal Femoral Resection on Ligament Balance in Total Knee Replacement. In Dorr LD (ed). The Knee: Papers of the First Scientific Meeting of the Knee Society. Baltimore, University Park Press 59–73, 1984.
22. Yoshii I, Whiteside LA, White SE, Milliano MT: Influence of prosthetic joint line position on knee kinematics and patellar position. J Arthroplasty 6:169–177, 1991.
23. Yoshioka Y, Siu D, Cooke TDV: The anatomy and functional axes of the femur. J Bone Joint Surg 69A:873–880, 1987.

Valgus Knee

5. Valgus Knee

Basic Principles

Ligament balancing in the valgus knee continues to challenge arthroplasty surgeons despite advances in instrumentation for bone resection and alignment. However, the application of basic principle alignment allows the surgeon to correct deformity and eliminate articular surface deficiencies by using reliable anatomic landmarks and axes of the femur and tibia to position the components. Using the central axis of the femur and tibia as a reference line for valgus angle ensures highly reproducible alignment in the frontal plane. Using the distal surface of the medial femoral condyle as the point of reference for distal femoral resection ensures that the distal surface of the femur will be in correct position relative to the medial ligaments and the patella. The anterior-posterior axis of the distal femur provides a reliable line of reference for rotational alignment of the femoral component so the patellar groove, intercondylar notch, and condylar surfaces are positioned correctly, and the epicondylar axis is aligned perpendicular to the mechanical axis of the femur and the long axis of the tibia in flexion and extension. Effective ligament balance relies entirely on this principle of first aligning the components correctly around these axes and positioning the femoral joint surfaces equidistant from the epicondylar axis throughout the arc of flexion. Extensive laboratory studies of kinematics and ligament function in the knee, and exhaustive clinical studies of ligament balancing during surgery and stability after surgery, consistently confirm that using the intact side of the deformed joint as a positioning reference for the joint surfaces throughout the flexion and extension arc provides surfaces around which the ligaments can be stabilized.

After correct alignment and positioning of the articular surfaces, a strategy is necessary to ensure correct ligament balance throughout the arc of flexion. Consideration of the functional effects of the lateral stabilizing structures in flexion and extension offers a basis from which to formulate this approach. A knee with contracture in the flexed and extended positions requires different procedures than one that is tight only in extension. A knee that is tight only in flexion also should be treated with different ligament release procedures than would be used for one with ligament contractures that appear only in the extended knee.

Ligaments that attach to the femur near the epicondyles, that is, near the axis through which the tibia rotates as the knee flexes and extends, function through the entire flexion arc of the knee. Those that attach to a point distant from the epicondylar axis function effectively only in full extension or in positions of fairly deep flexion. On the lateral side of the knee the structures attaching to the femur near the epicondyle are the lateral collateral ligament, the popliteus tendon, and the posterolateral corner capsule. The lateral collateral ligament is a stabilizing structure in flexion and extension, and has rotational and varus stabilizing effects. The popliteus tendon complex also has passive varus stabilizing effects in flexion and extension, but has a more prominent role in external rotational stabilization of the tibia on the femur. The posterolateral corner has primary stabilizing effects in extension, but also is effective in flexion. These three structures are appropriate to release for a knee that is excessively tight laterally in flexion and extension. The iliotibial band is attached at a point above the knee far from the epicondylar axis, so it is aligned perpendicular to the joint surface when the knee is extended. It can contribute to lateral knee stability in this position, but when the knee is flexed to 90°, it is parallel to the joint surface, and cannot stabilize the knee to varus stress. The lateral posterior capsular structures are tight only in full extension, and are slack when the knee is flexed. Release of either the lateral posterior capsule or the iliotibial band is appropriate only for a knee that is tight laterally in extension, and would have little effect on lateral knee stability in the flexed position.

In the valgus knee, deficiency of the lateral femoral condyle distorts the normal relationships of the mechanical axes, and restoration of normal alignment must precede ligament balancing. Awareness of these principles provides a rational plan for ligament releases in the valgus knee after total knee arthroplasty.

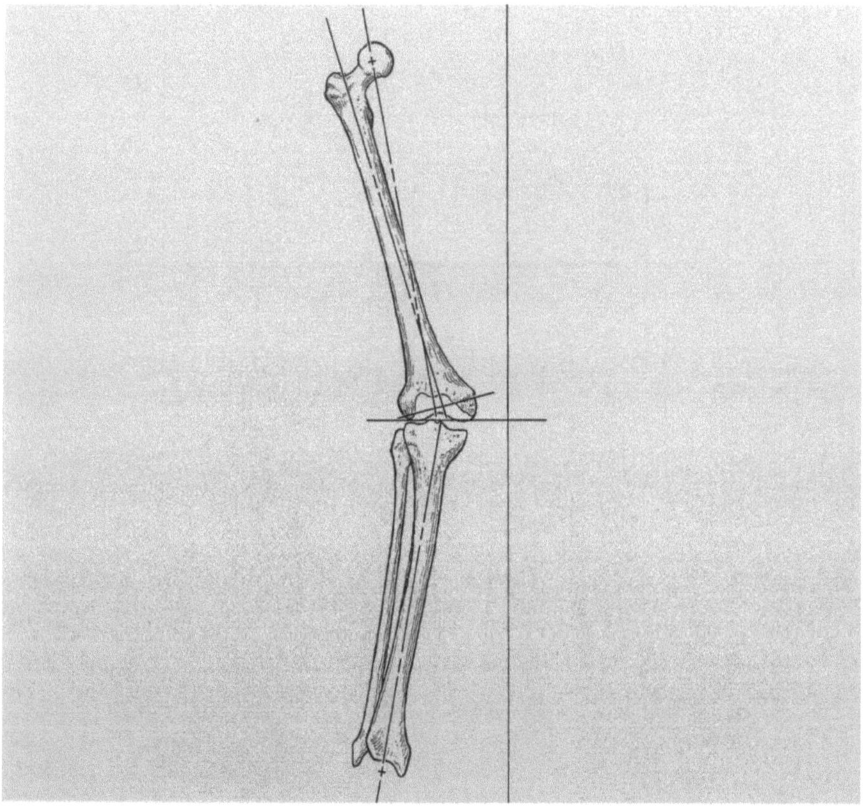

Fig. 108. In the valgus knee the lateral femoral condyle is deficient, usually distally and posteriorly, so the knee is in valgus both in the extended and flexed positions. A valgus curvature usually exists in the mid-shaft of the femur and tibia, so that the line down the midshaft diaphyseal medullary canal crosses the joint medial to the center. Entry points into the joint for intramedullary alignment rods should be medialized 5mm-10mm to accommodate and correct this valgus curvature.

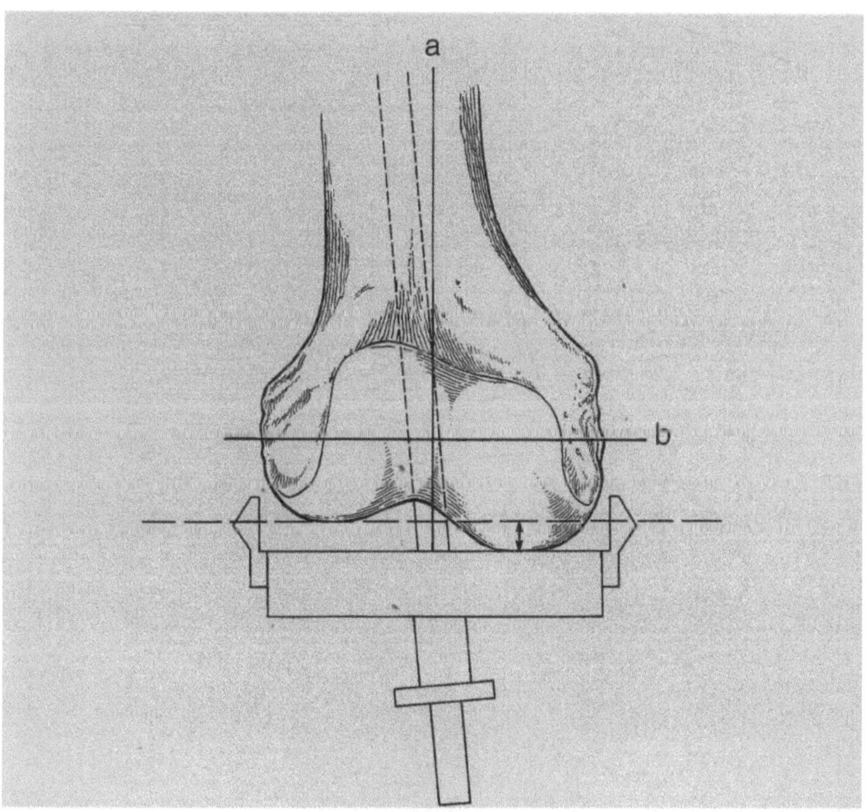

Fig. 109. The intramedullary alignment rod lies slightly medial to the center of the patellar groove, and the cutting guide is set at a 5° valgus angle. This will align the joint surface perpendicular to the mechanical axis of the femur (a), and parallel to the epicondylar axis (b). The cutting guide seats against the high (medial) side, which is the reference for resection of the joint surfaces. The thickness of the implant is resected distally from the medial side. In some cases resection of the thickness of the implant from the medial side results in minimal or no resection from the lateral side of the distal femur. Regardless of the lateral bone deficit, the medial should be used as the reference surface, and augmentation of the lateral surface should be done to make up for the deficit.

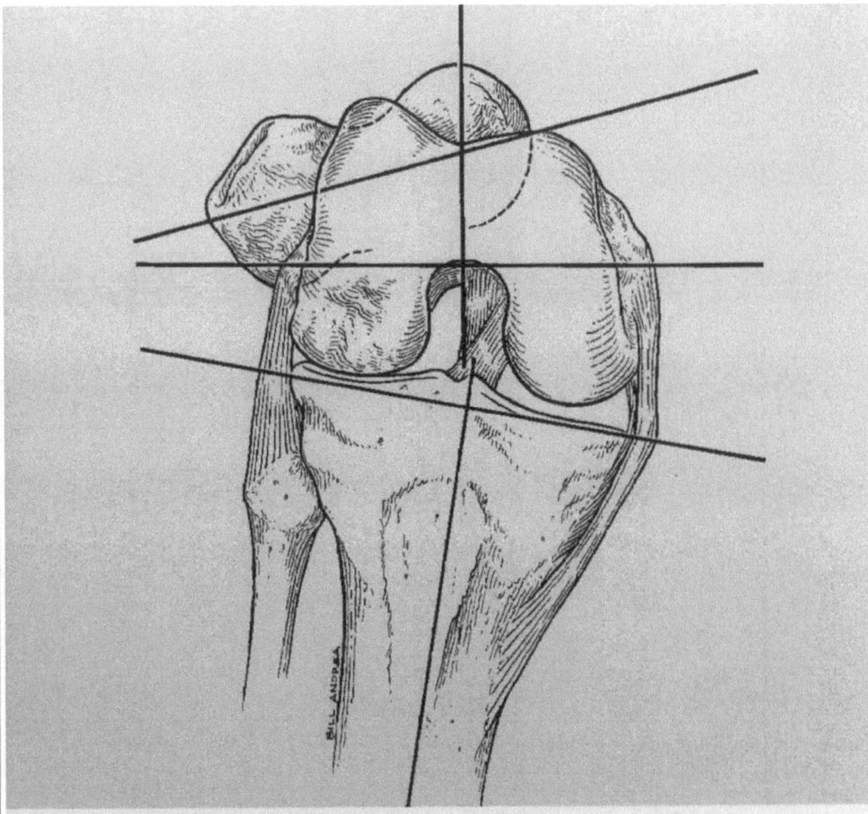

Fig. 110. Viewed from the distal end, the femur usually can be seen to have deficiency of the posterior lateral femoral condylar surfaces. The anterior-posterior axis is especially helpful for orientation of varus-valgus alignment of the valgus knee in flexion. The anterior-posterior axis, constructed from the center of the intercondylar notch posteriorly through the deepest part of the patellar groove, is perpen-dicular to the epicondylar axis, and passes through the center of the femoral head. If osteophytes obscure the edges of the intercondylar notch, the lateral edge of the posterior cruciate ligament serves as a reliable landmark for the center of the notch. The long axis of the tibia is no longer collinear with the anterior-posterior axis of the femur, but is angled toward valgus as it is in full extension.

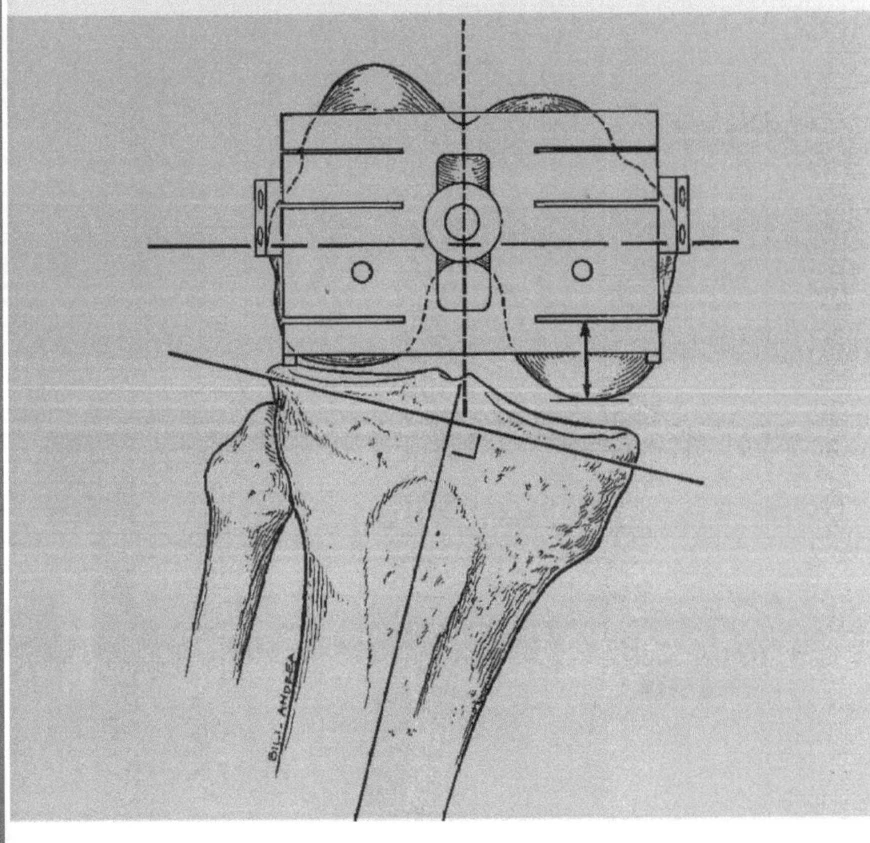

Fig. 111. The cutting guide for femoral resection is aligned so the surfaces are resected perpendicular to the anterior-posterior axis of the femur (a) and parallel with the epicondylar axis (b), resecting the thickness of the implant from the intact medial femoral condyle (arrow), and much less from the deficient lateral side. This places the joint surfaces in anatomic position to correct the valgus position in flexion, and places the patellar groove correctly with the mechanical axis of the lower extremity. The tibial surface is resected perpendicular to the long axis of the tibia. The lateral ligaments are still tight, and the tibia is held in valgus malalignment by the ligament contractures.

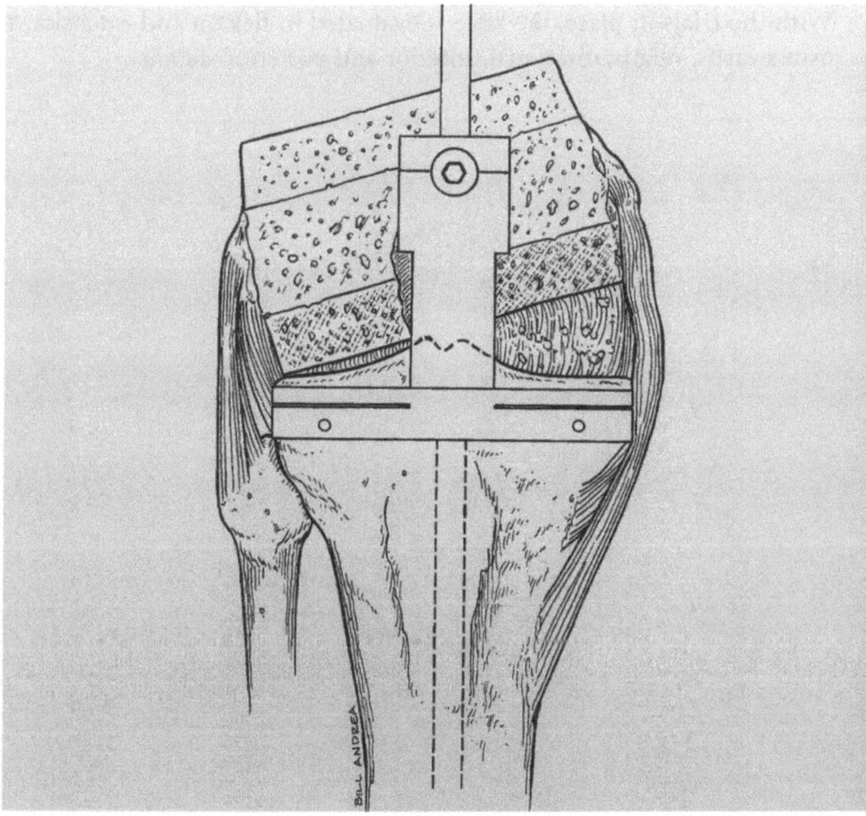

Fig. 112. After the femoral surfaces are resected and the resected pieces removed, the tibial surface is resected perpendicular to the long axis of the tibia in the coronal plane, and sloped 4°–7° posteriorly in the sagittal plane. As is done for the femur, the thickness of the implant is resected from the intact side. Usually there is minimal bone deficiency on the surface of the tibia.

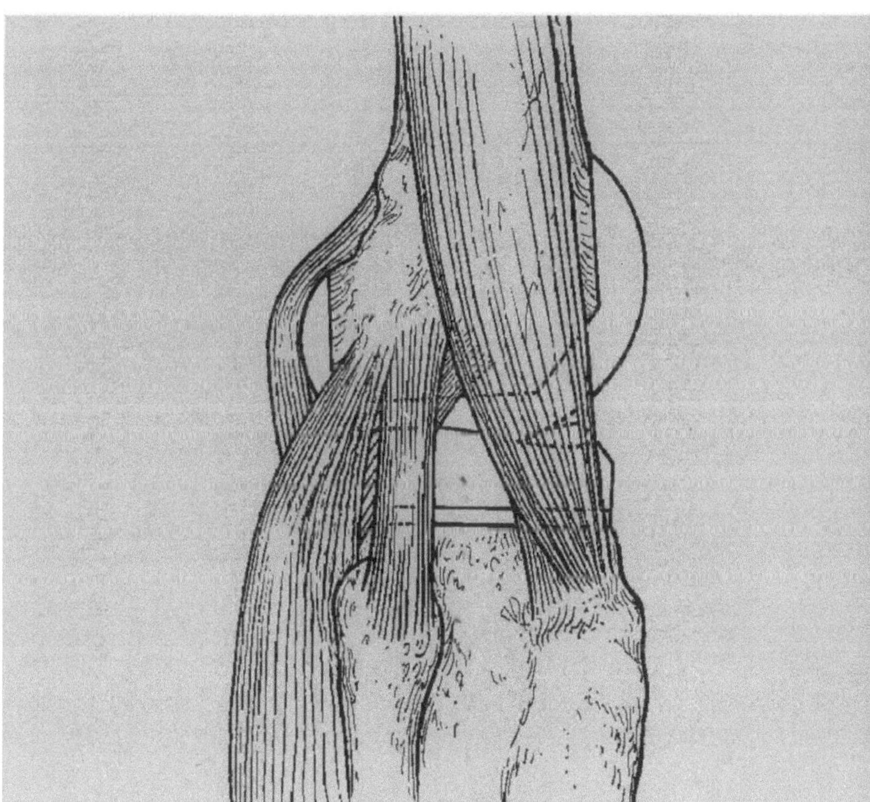

Fig. 113. Next the trials are inserted and stability is evaluated in flexion and extension. The lateral collateral ligament, popliteus tendon, and the posterolateral corner fibrous capsule are attached to the femur near the center of rotation of the tibia, so they have an effect both in flexion and extension. The lateral collateral ligament and posterolateral corner are more effective in extension, and the popliteus tendon is more effective in flexion, but they both have some effect throughout the flexion arc. The posterolateral corner capsular tissue is densely bound to the lateral gastro-cnemius tendon, and is effective mostly in extension. The iliotibial band and posterior capsule are effective only in extension as valgus stabilizers.

With the trials in place, the knee is evaluated in flexion and extension to assess varus, valgus, rotational, anterior and posterior stability.

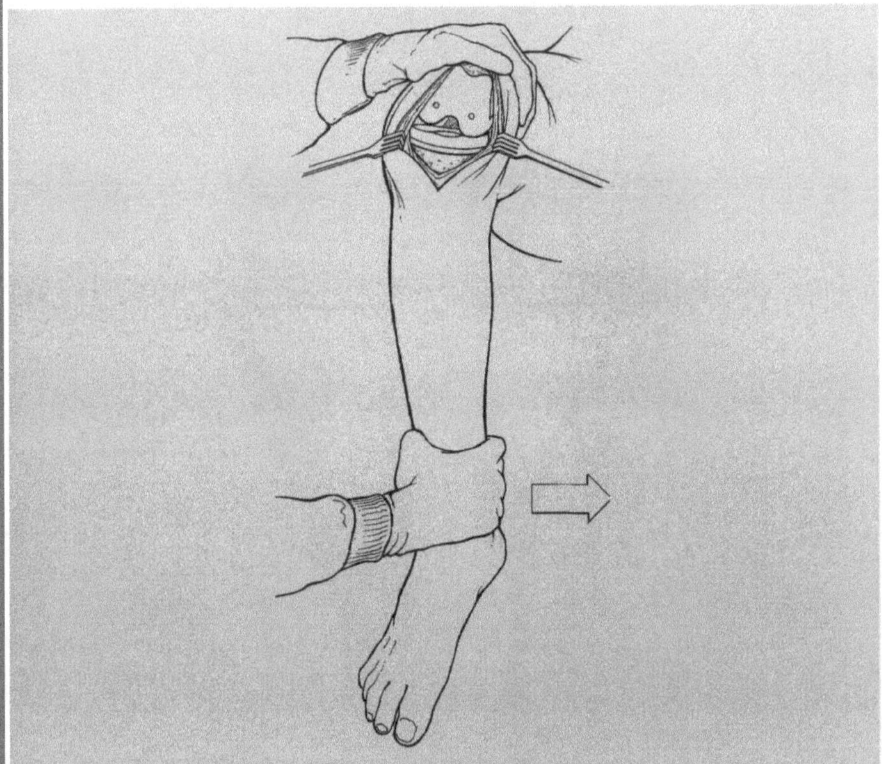

Fig. 114. The knee is evaluated in flexion and extension to assess varus, valgus, rotational, anterior, and posterior stability. To test the knee in flexion, the ankle is grasped with one hand while the other hand steadies the knee.

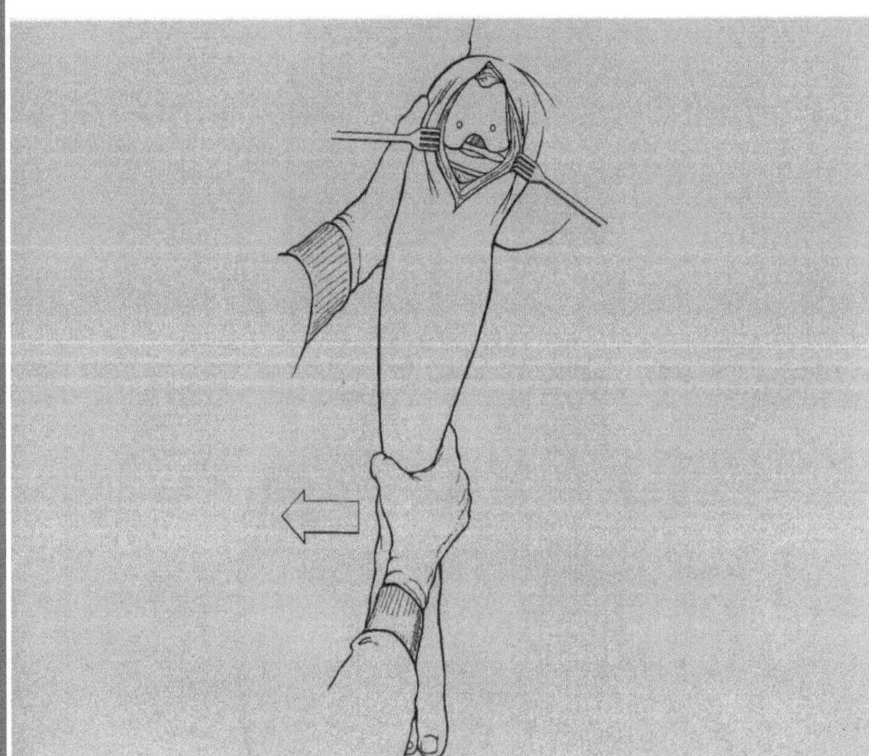

Fig. 115. The extremity then is rotated internally through the hip until the medial ligaments are stressed, then rotated externally until the lateral ligaments are stressed.

5.1. Tight Laterally Flexion and Extension

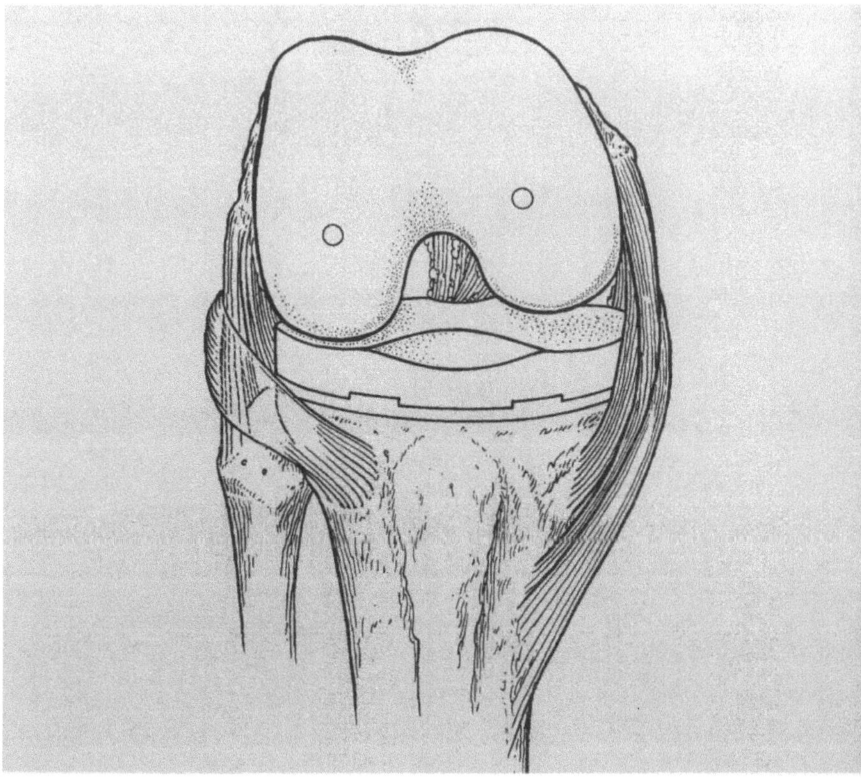

Fig. 116. In this case the knee is tight laterally and gapes medially. It also pivots around the lateral ligament structures. This indicates that either the lateral collateral ligament or popliteus complex, or both, are tight. Nothing can be determined yet about knee stability in extension.

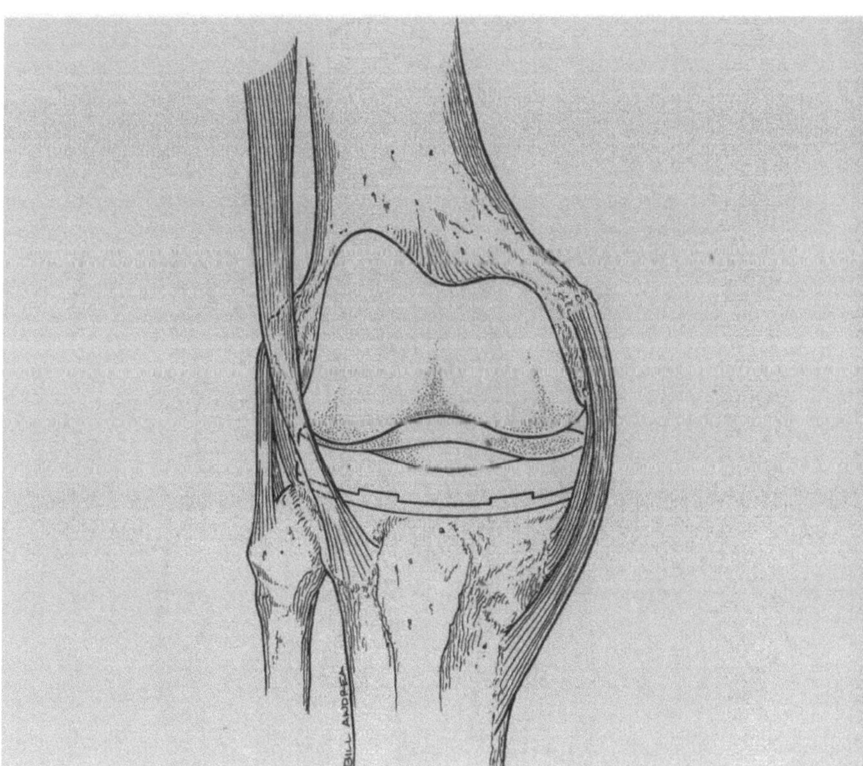

Fig. 117. Next the knee is extended and the varus-valgus, rotational, and anterior-posterior stability tests are repeated. In this case the knee is tight laterally and loose medially. The lateral collateral ligament, popliteus tendon, iliotibial band, and lateral posterior capsule all may be involved in causing excessive tightening laterally in the extended position. It is already known from the flexion stability tests that the lateral collateral ligament, popliteus tendon, posterolateral corner, or all three are tight. In fact, these three structures which attach near the femoral epicondyle may be the only tight structures in the knee, so addressing the tightness in flexion should be done first since release of the iliotibial band and posterior capsule may not be necessary.

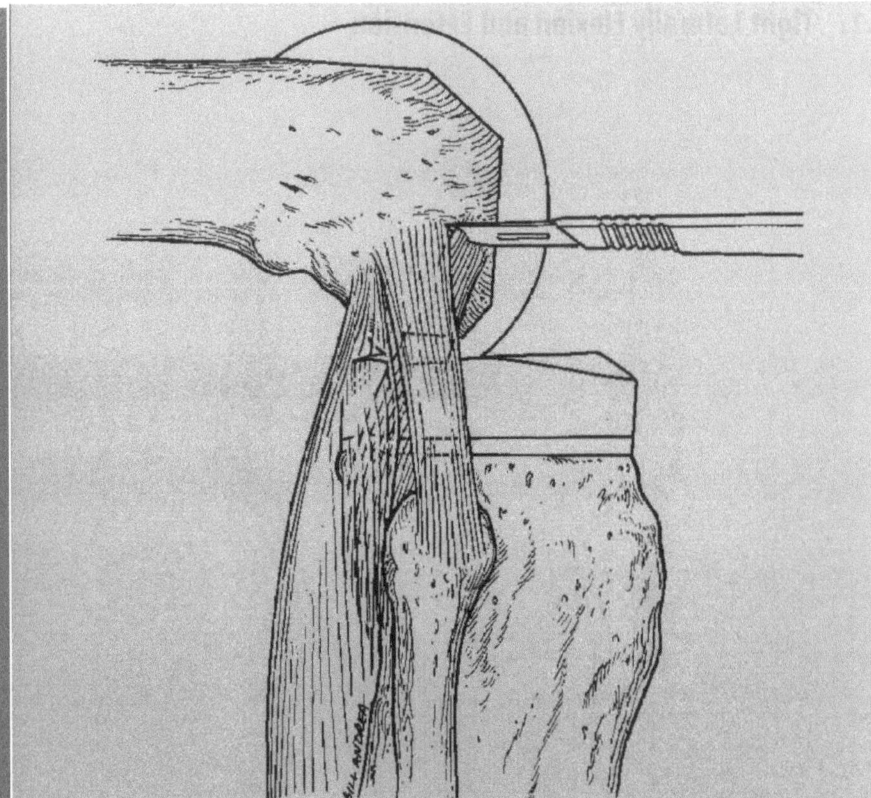

Fig. 118. To release the lateral epicondylar structures, the knee is flexed to 90°. The popliteus tendon is released directly from the femur, and allowed to retract.

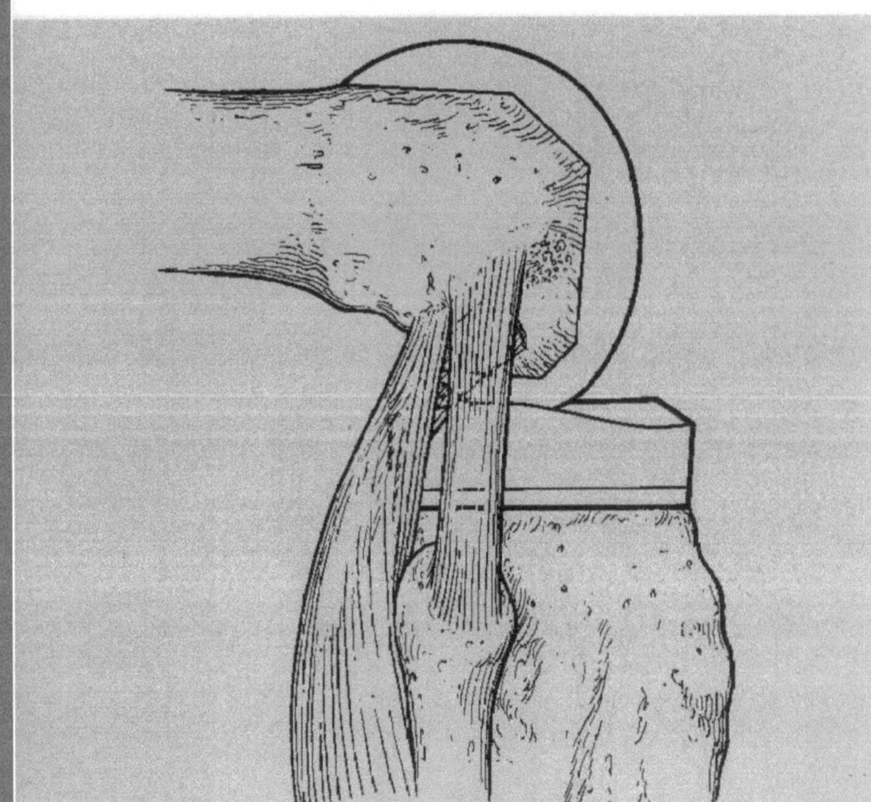

Fig. 119. Because of its secondary attachments to the capsule and lateral collateral ligament, the popliteus tendon retracts only about 5mm–10mm. The knee should be tested again to evaluate the effect of release of the popliteus tendon. If the knee is still tight on the lateral side in flexion, the lateral collateral ligament should be released, also directly from its bone attachment, leaving intact the capsular attachments just behind it. If this is not sufficient, the posterolateral corner capsule is released.

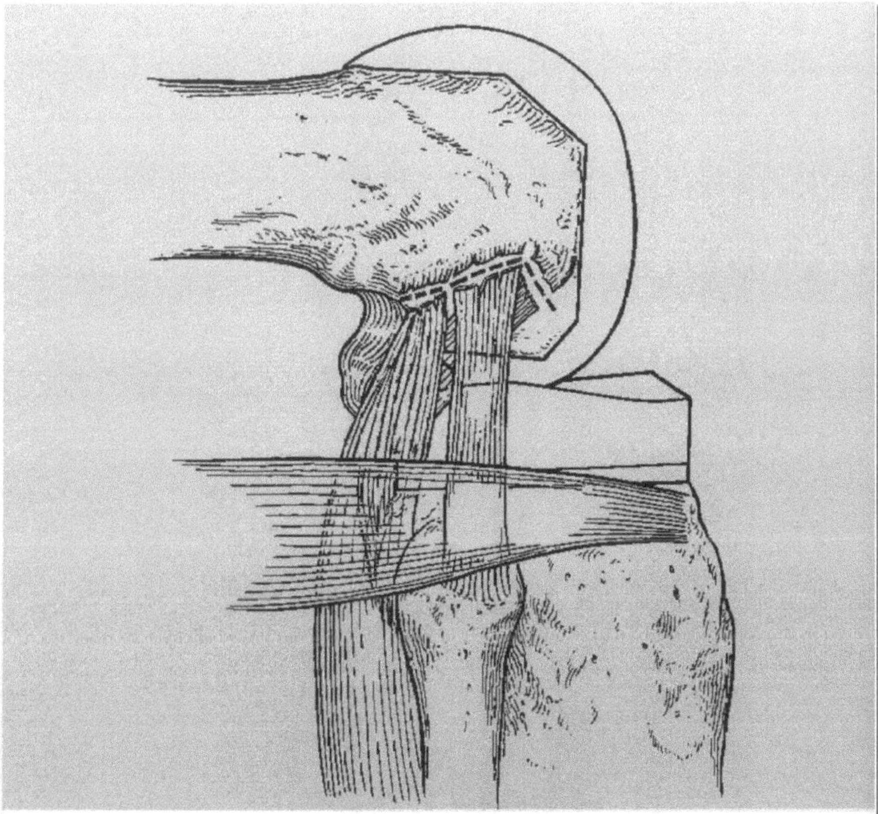

Fig. 120. Now that the lateral collateral ligament, popliteus tendon, and postero-lateral corner have been released, they retract partially, but remain attached to the surrounding capsule and dense overlying synovial membrane, and so continue to function as lateral stabilizers. Release of the popliteus tendon, lateral collateral ligament, and rarely the postero lateral corner capsule always corrects lateral ligament tension in flexion because these are the only structures that stabilize the lateral side of the knee in flexion. The iliotibial band and posterior capsule remain as stabilizers in extension, and may still apply deforming forces, but only in the extended knee.

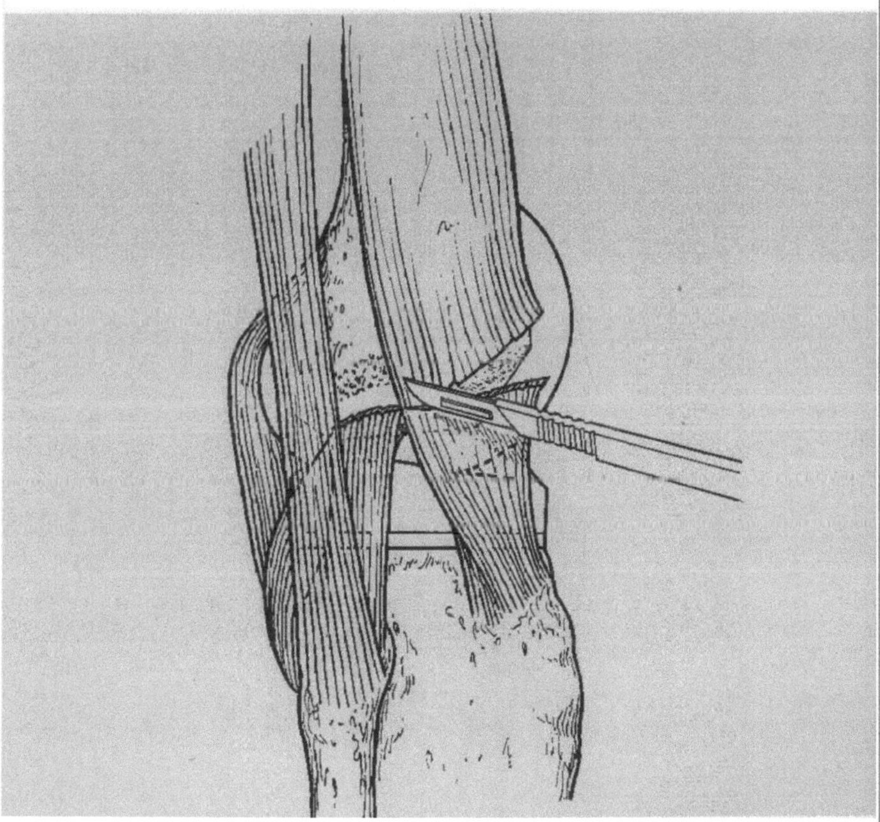

Fig. 121. If the knee remains tight laterally in extension, the iliotibial band should be released. In this case the release is done just above the joint line, extrasynovially so that the iliotibial band elongates, but remains attached to the synovial membrane, and can continue to support the lateral side of the knee in extension. The posterior cruciate ligament, posterior capsule, and biceps femoris remain as lateral stabilizers in extension.

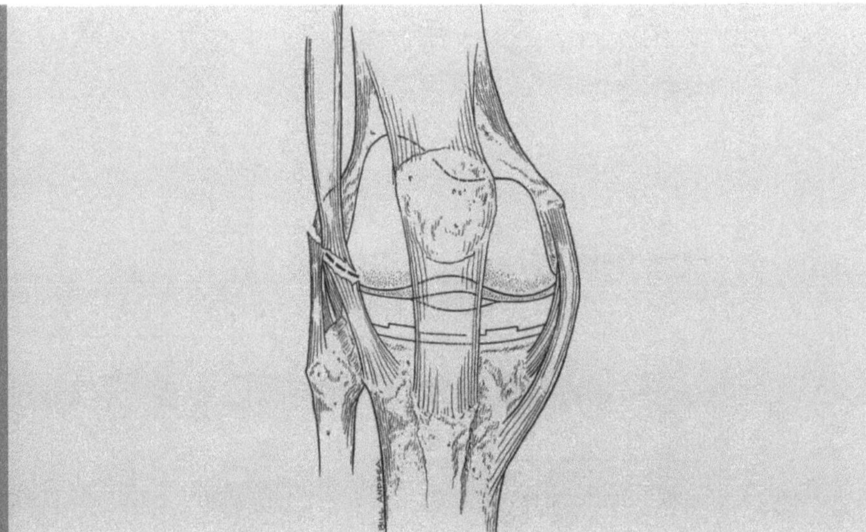

Fig. 122. The knee now is balanced in flexion and extension, but is likely to be loose both medially and laterally due to medial ligament stretching and lateral ligament release. In rare cases the knee remains tight laterally in extension, and requires release of the lateral posterior capsule, the last remaining lateral ligamentous structure.

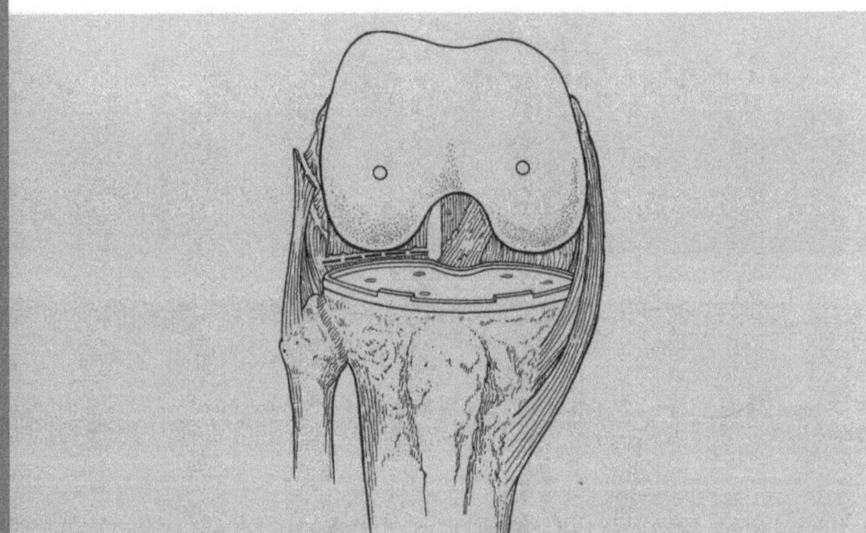

Fig. 123. When the posterior capsule must be released, access is achieved by removing the tibial spacer and distracting the joint with the knee flexed 90°. The capsule either can be transected at the joint line or released from the posterior surface of the femur with a curved osteotome as illustrated in figure 133. Release of the posterior lateral capsule from the tibia should not be done because of damage of the damaging the peroneal nerve.

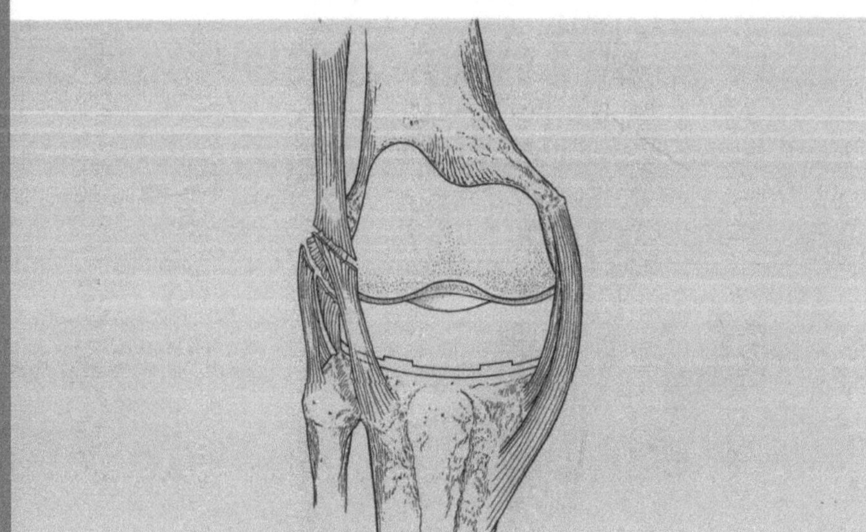

Fig. 124. A thicker tibial spacer has been added to tension the medial ligaments. The lateral ligaments have been lengthened to match the medial structures in flexion and extension.

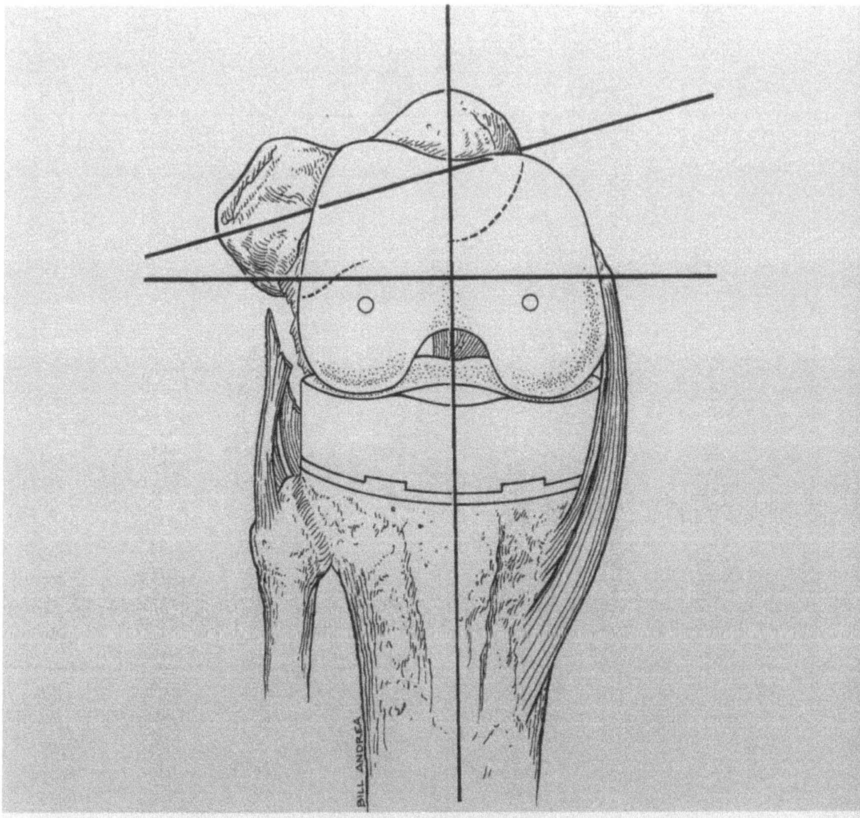

Fig. 125. In flexion the ligaments remain well balanced, and are tensioned appropriately by the thicker spacer. The anterior-posterior axis now passes through the center of the femoral head, and aligns precisely with the long axis of the tibia.

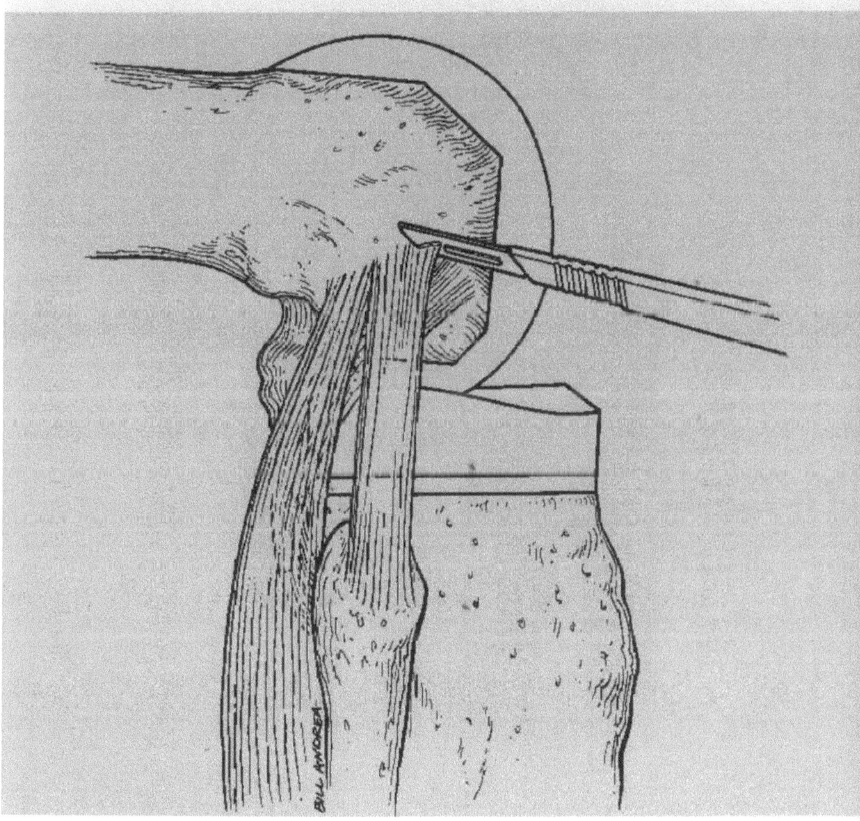

Fig. 126. Occasionally a knee is found to be tight on the lateral side in flexion and extension, but more so in extension. The lateral collateral ligament is most effective in extension, and the popliteus tendon is most effective in flexion. So in cases similar to this illustration, only the lateral collateral ligament is released. This release is done with a knife, detaching the ligament directly from the bone, but leaving it attached to the surrounding capsule and popliteus tendon.

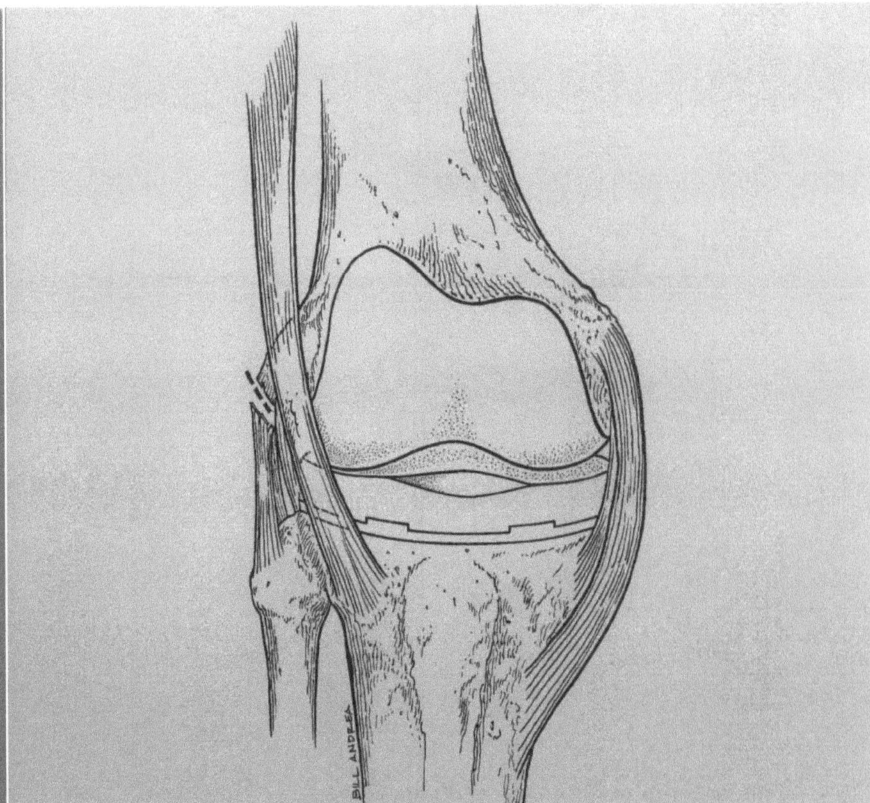

Fig. 127. In extension the knee is still supported laterally by the iliotibial band, posterior capsule, the popliteus tendon, and the posterolateral corner.

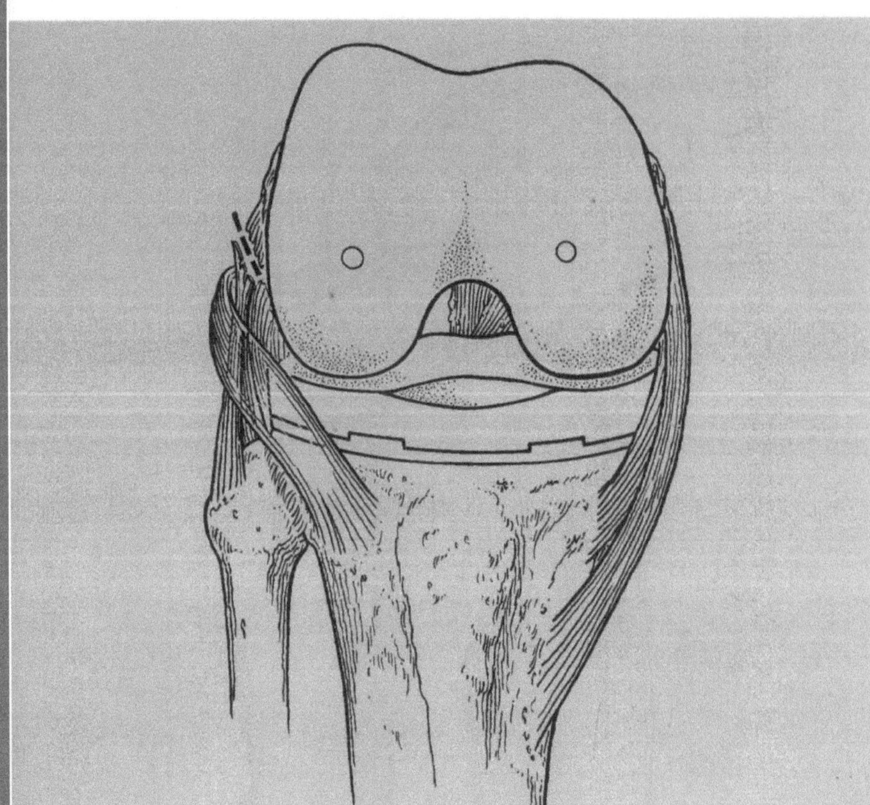

Fig. 128. In flexion the lateral collateral ligament release has less effect because the lateral collateral ligament normally is somewhat slack in the flexed position. The popliteus tendon, posterolateral corner, and posterior cruciate ligament continue to provide lateral stability in flexion.

5.2. Tight Laterally in Extension, Normal Stability in Flexion

Occasionally, after correct bone resection and insertion of trial implants, it is apparent that the knee is balanced in flexion, but it is tight on the lateral side in extension only.

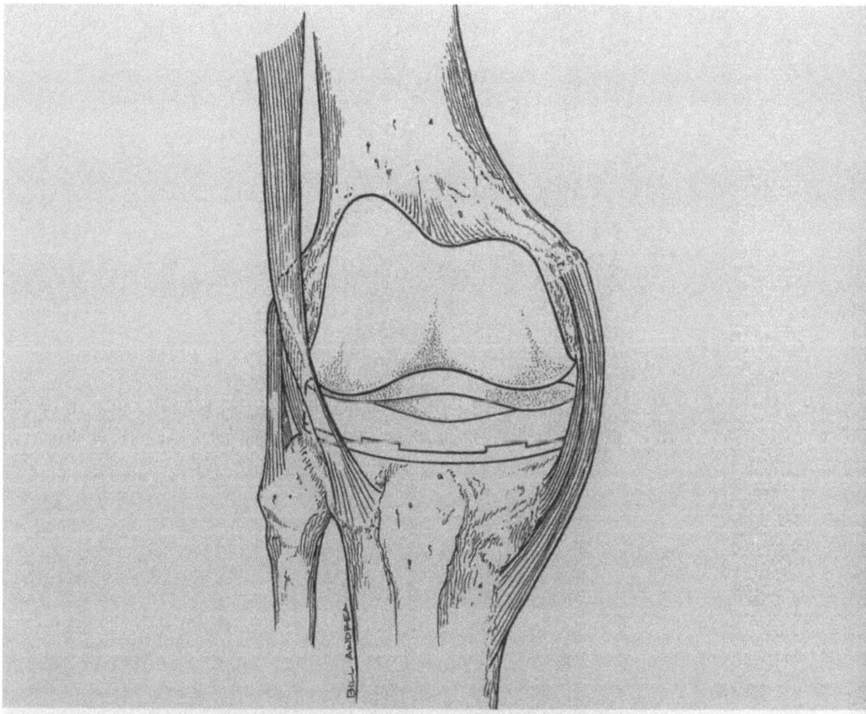

Fig. 129. After correct bone resection and insertion of the trial components, the knee is tight laterally in extension, and spontaneously gapes medially. The tight iliotibial band tends to externally rotate the tibia.

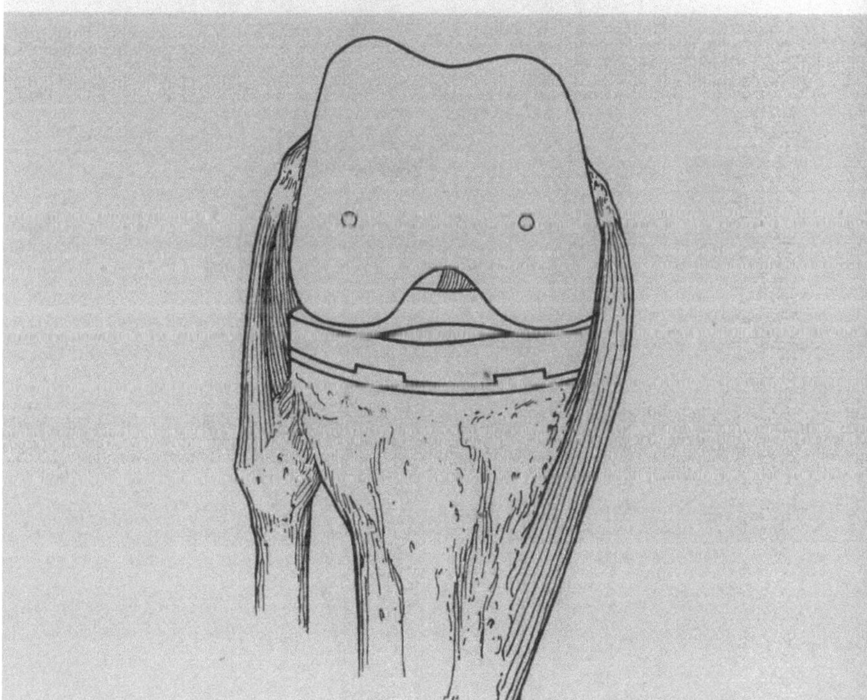

Fig. 130. With the knee flexed 90°, the joint surfaces seat normally and the joint opens normally medially and laterally with valgus and varus stress.

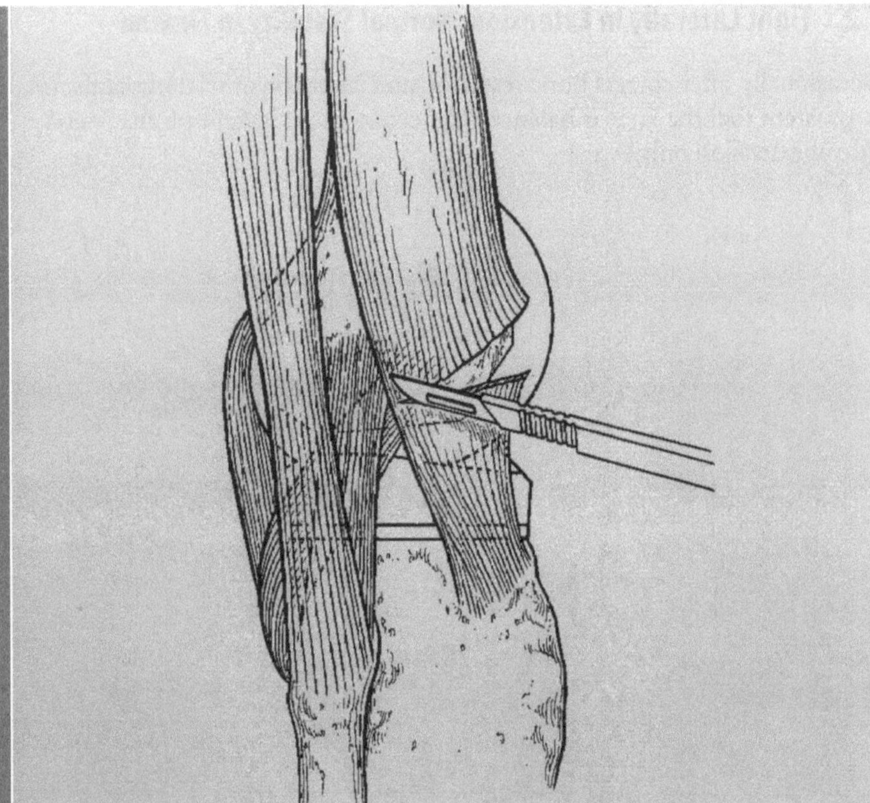

Fig. 131. The initial step in correcting the knee that is tight laterally in extension only is to release the iliotibial band. A knife is used to transect the iliotibial band from front-to-back, leaving the synovial membrane intact. The posterior capsule and biceps femoris tendon also may be tight, and may leave the joint in need of further correction.

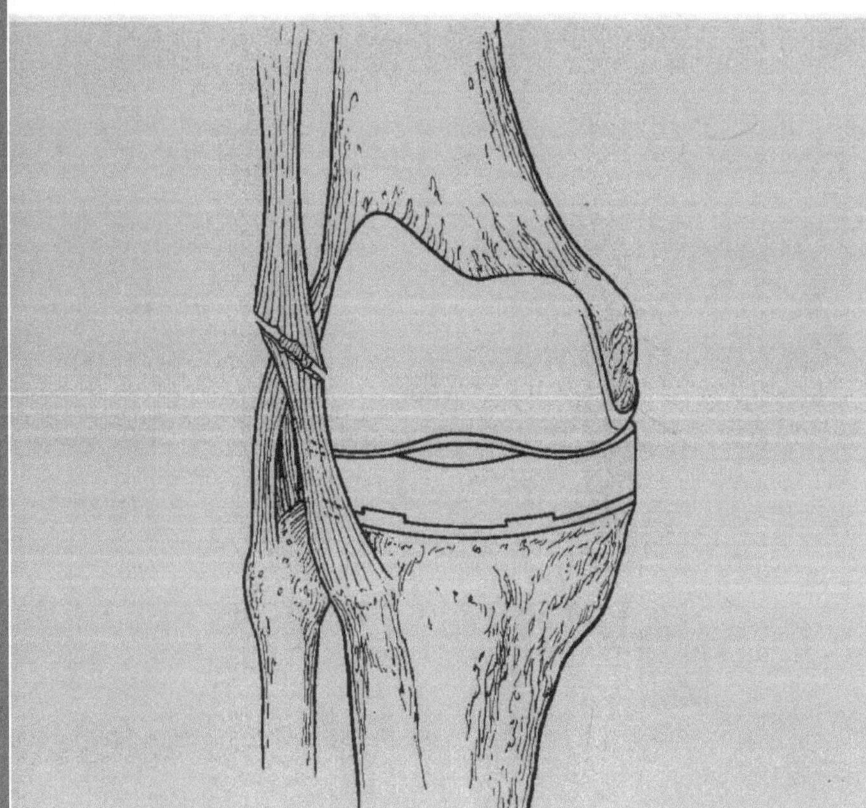

Fig. 132. Now the knee no longer gapes spontaneously medially in full extension, and the tendency for the tibia to rotate externally has been corrected.

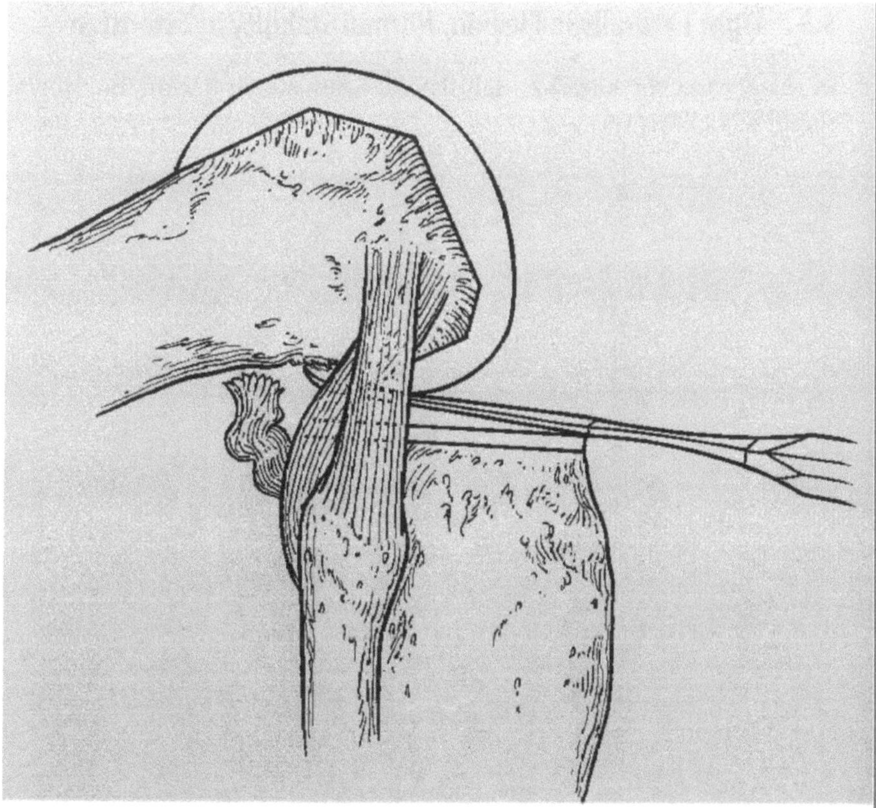

Fig. 133. In a few cases the knee remains tight laterally only in full extension after release of the iliotibial band. In these cases the lateral posterior capsule is the next structure to be released. The lateral posterior capsule is released by removing the polyethylene spacer and inserting the curved osteotome behind the knee against the femoral attachment of the posterior capsule, then gently tapping the end of the osteotome. This release does not affect stability of the lateral side of the knee in flexion.

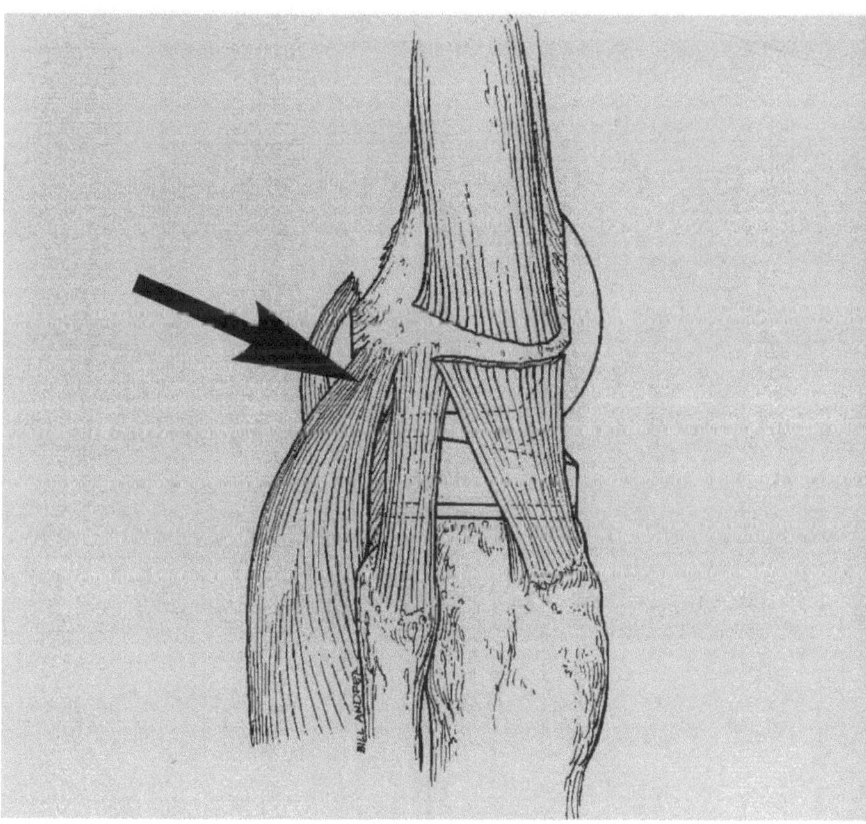

Fig. 134. Now the knee is correctly stabilized in extension. The lateral collateral ligament, popliteus tendon, and posterior cruciate ligament maintain lateral stability. In rare cases, further release in extension is necessary, and the postero-lateral corner capsule is released (arrow).

5.3. Tight Laterally in Flexion, Normal Stability in Extension

In many cases the knee has tight lateral ligaments in flexion, but normal stability in extension.

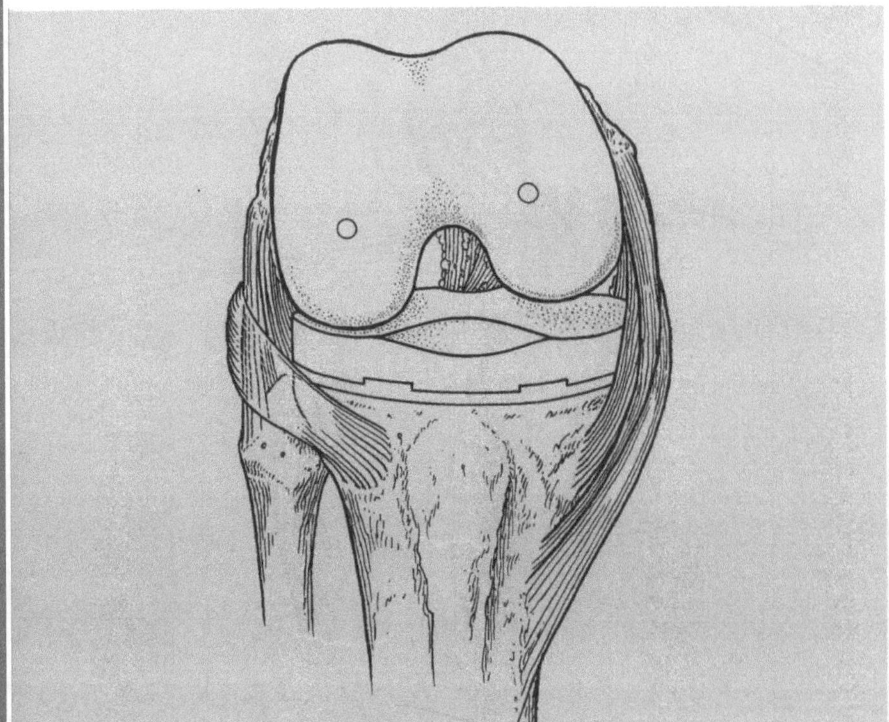

Fig. 135. In the case illustrated here, the knee opens 4–5mm with valgus stress, but does not open at all to varus stress.

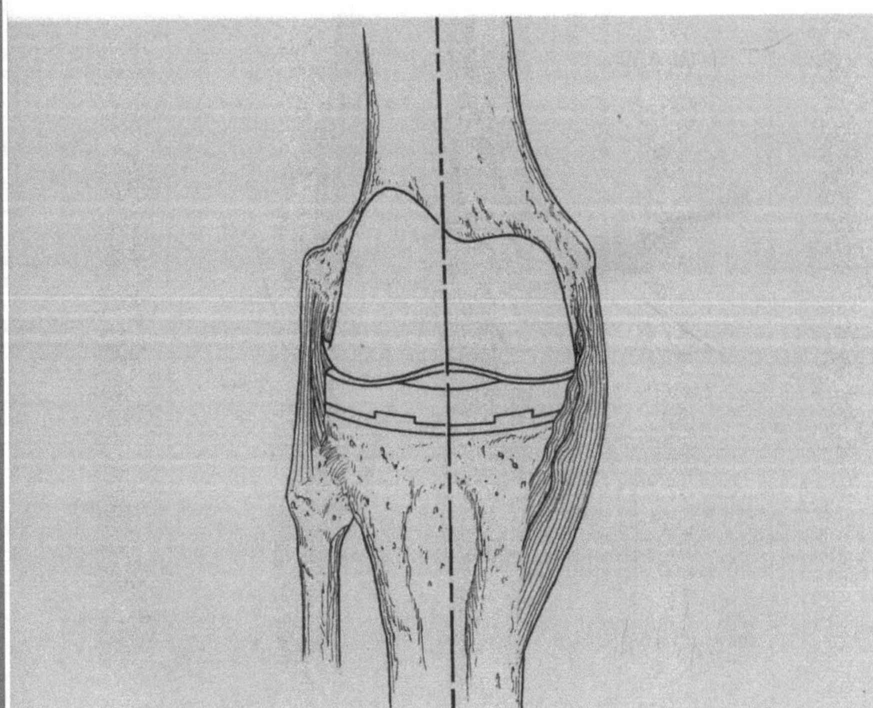

Fig. 136. In full extension the knee has normal medial and lateral stability.

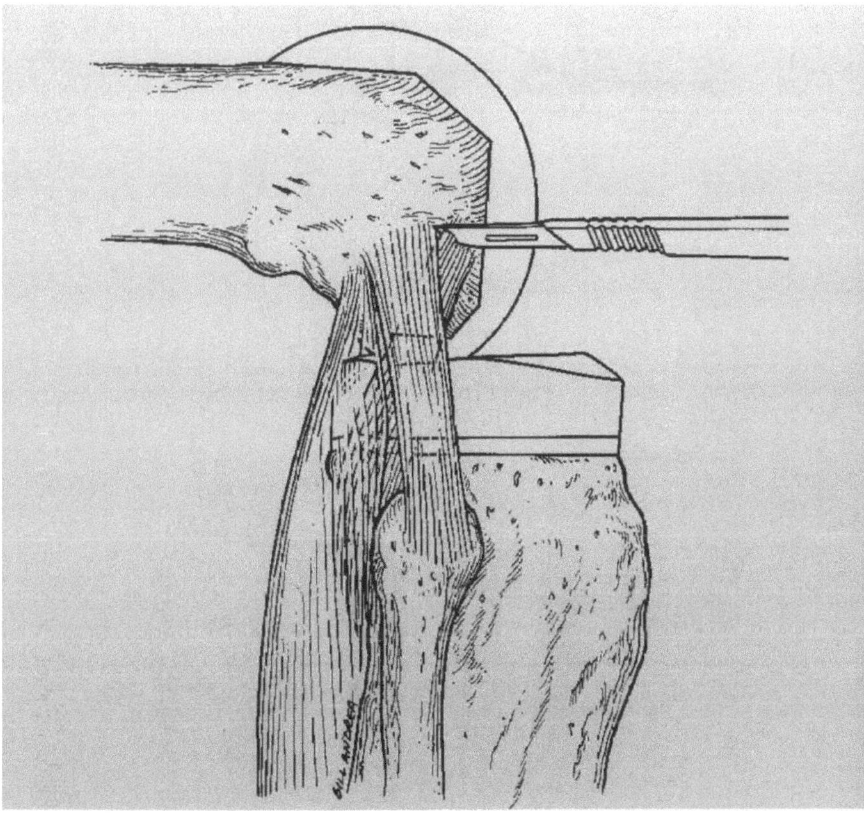

Fig. 137. Because the popliteus tendon is more effective in flexion than in extension, it is released first. This is done with a knife, releasing the fibers directly from their attachments to bone, leaving the tendon attached to the surrounding synovial membrane, capsule, and lateral collateral ligament.

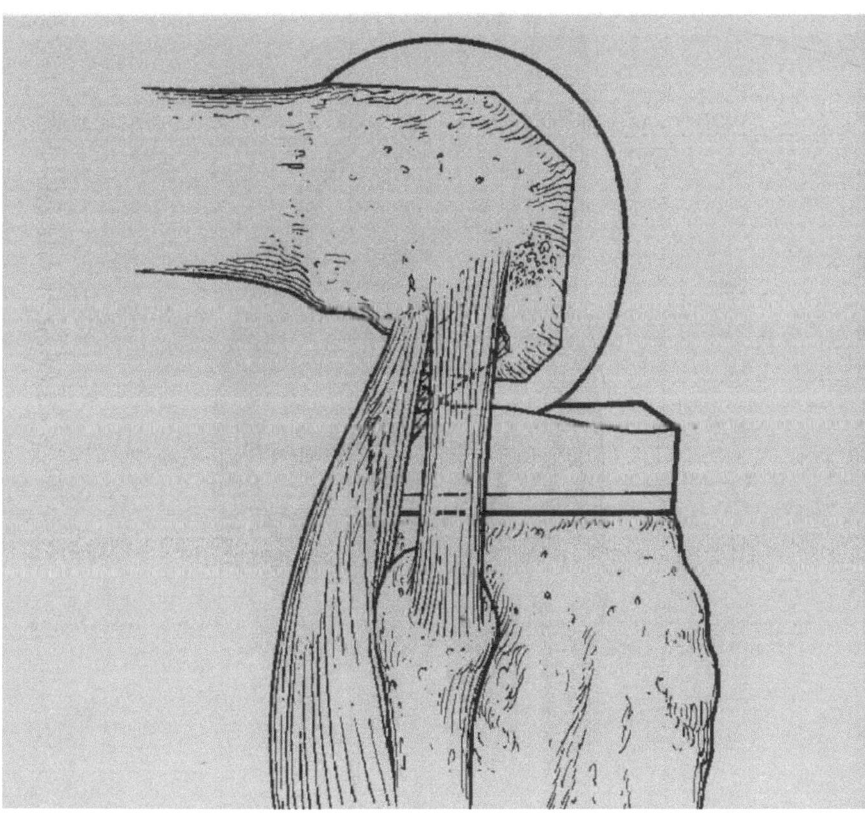

Fig. 138. The popliteus tendon slides distally 5–10mm, but remains functional as a lateral stabilizing structure. The knee should be tested again, and if release is not sufficient to achieve correct lateral laxity in flexion, the lateral collateral ligament, and finally the posterolateral corner should be released.

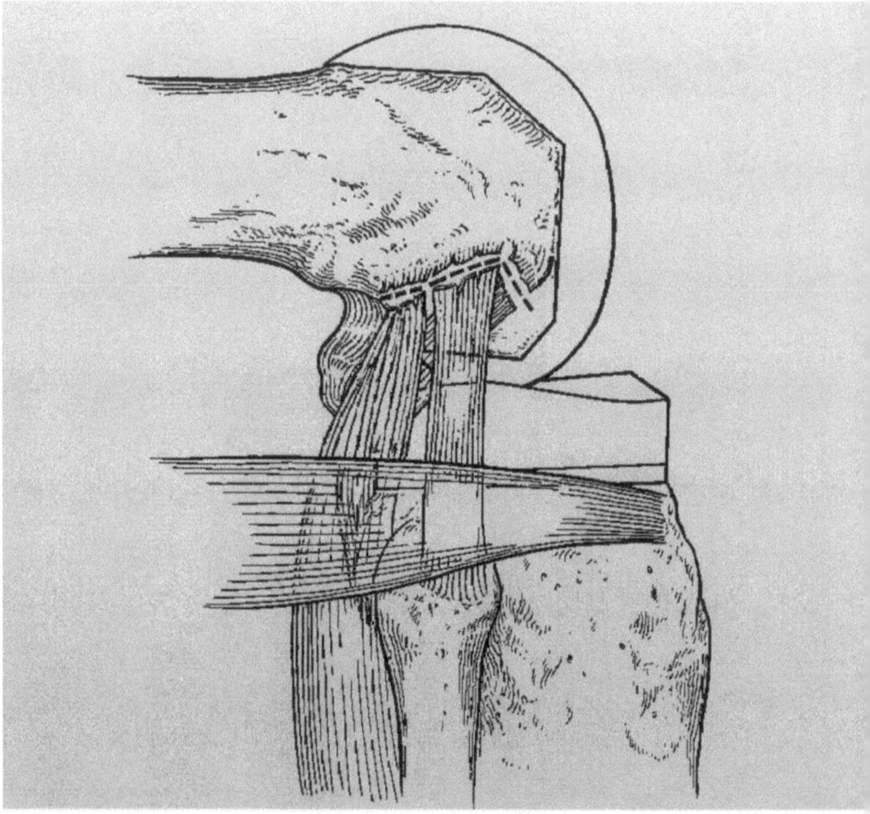

Fig. 139. As with the popliteus tendon, the lateral collateral ligament and posterolateral corner are released directly from their attachments to the lateral femoral condyle, but they remain attached to the surrounding dense fibrous capsule and synovial membrane. Because these structures are the only ones that stabilize the lateral side of the knee in flexion, this release always corrects the lateral ligament contracture in flexion.

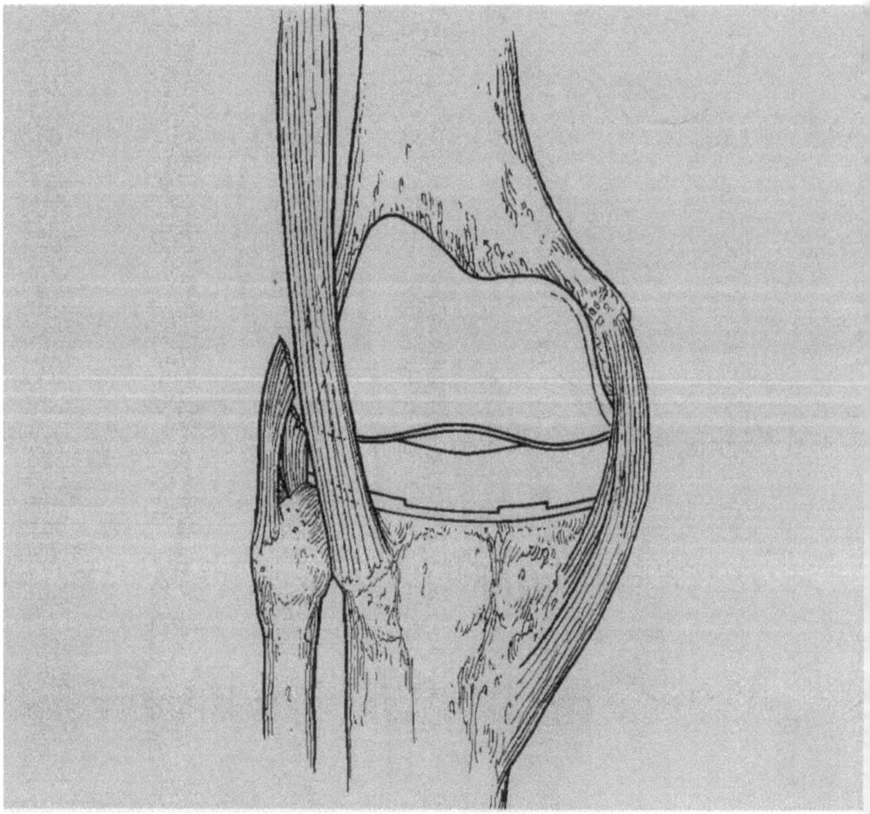

Fig. 140. In full extension the knee is stabilized by the iliotibial band and lateral posterior capsule.

5.4. Deficient Posterior Cruciate Ligament

Because the posterior cruciate ligament is a medial structure, it often is stretched and deficient in the valgus knee. Because the popliteus tendon and lateral collateral ligament are secondary posterior stabilizing structures, the valgus knee often is unstable posteriorly after ligament balancing.

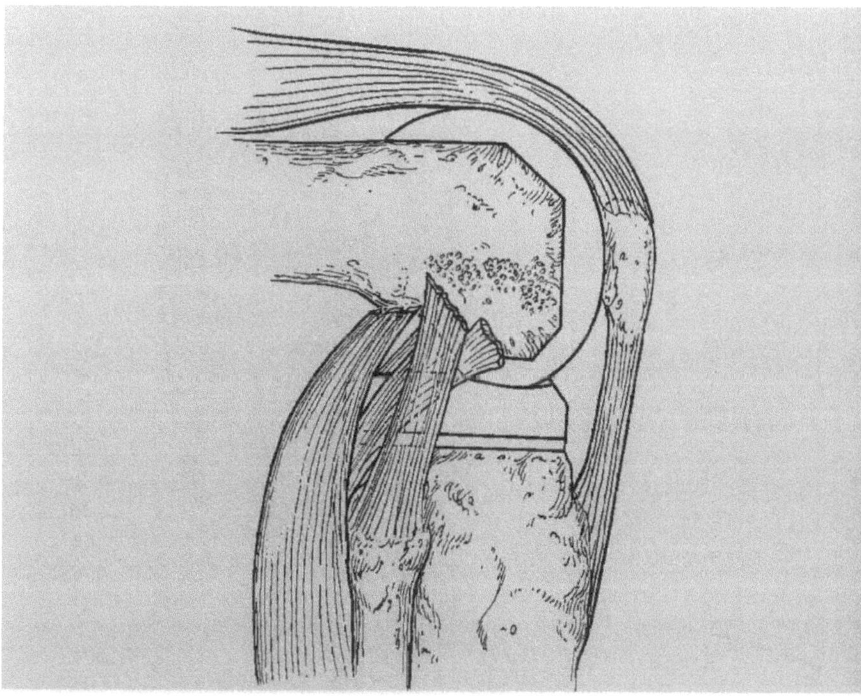

Fig. 141. The posterior cruciate ligament often is deficient in the valgus knee, so after complete release of the lateral collateral ligament, popliteus tendon, and posterolateral corner, the tibia may sag posteriorly. This places the quadriceps at a disadvantage.

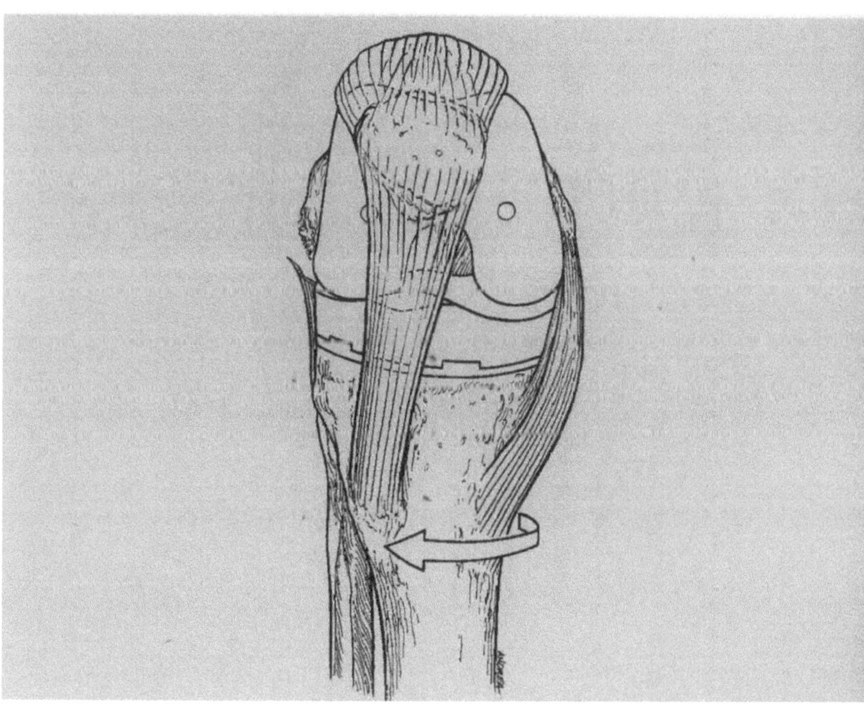

Fig. 142. Loss of the external rotational stabilizing effect of the lateral collateral ligament, popliteus tendon, and posterolateral corner capsule allows the tibia to rotate externally under load bearing, and can cause lateral tracking of the patella.

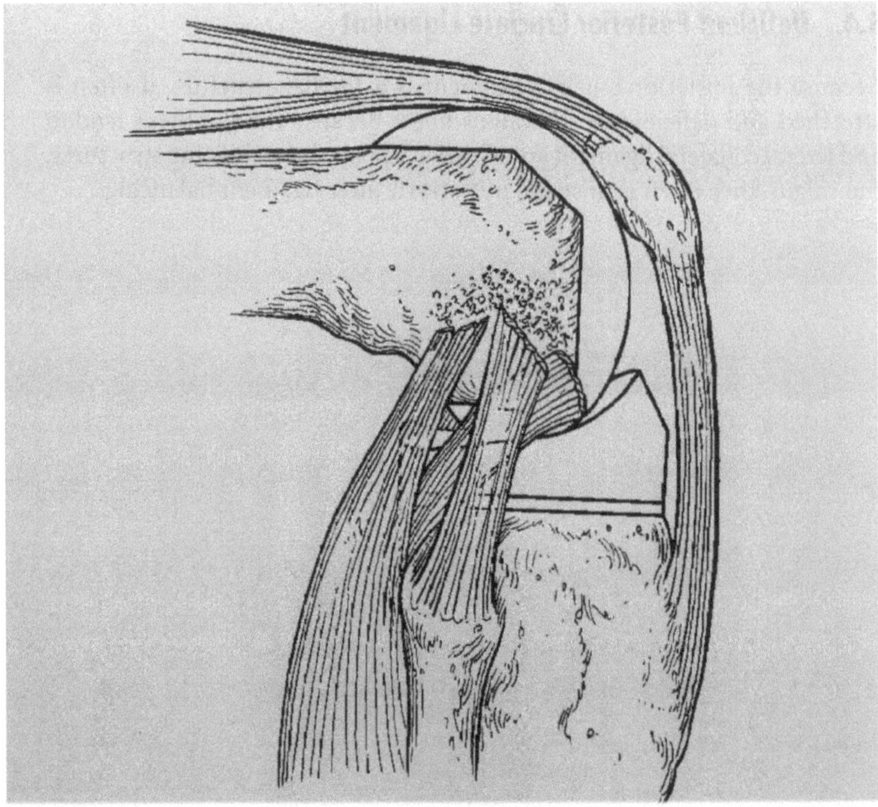

Fig. 143. The conforming plus polyethylene component holds the tibia forward, and improves the quadriceps advantage.

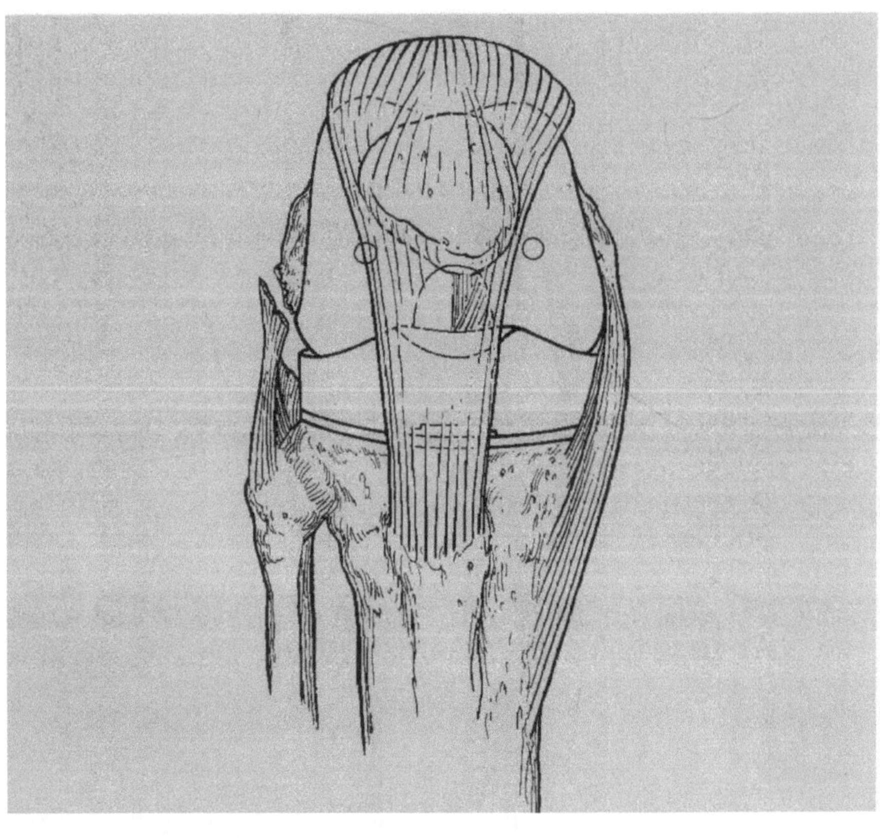

Fig. 144. The conforming plus polyethylene component also provides rotational stabilization, centralizing the tibial tubercle and quadriceps complex.

5.5. Pitfalls of the Valgus Knee

5.5.1. Release of Extension-only Stabilizers -Tight in Flexion and Extension

One of the most common mistakes made when correcting the valgus knee is to release extension-only stabilizing structures first in a knee that is tight laterally both in flexion and extension. Such a knee has tight lateral structures in flexion, so release of the lateral collateral ligament and popliteus tendon definitely will be necessary, and may correct the entire knee in flexion and extension. Release of the extension-only structures may not be necessary. Early release of the iliotibial band and posterior capsule will not correct the lateral contracture in flexion, and after release of the lateral collateral ligament and popliteus tendon, may leave the knee too loose in extension.

5.5.2. Release of Extension-only Structures -Tight in Flexion and Extension

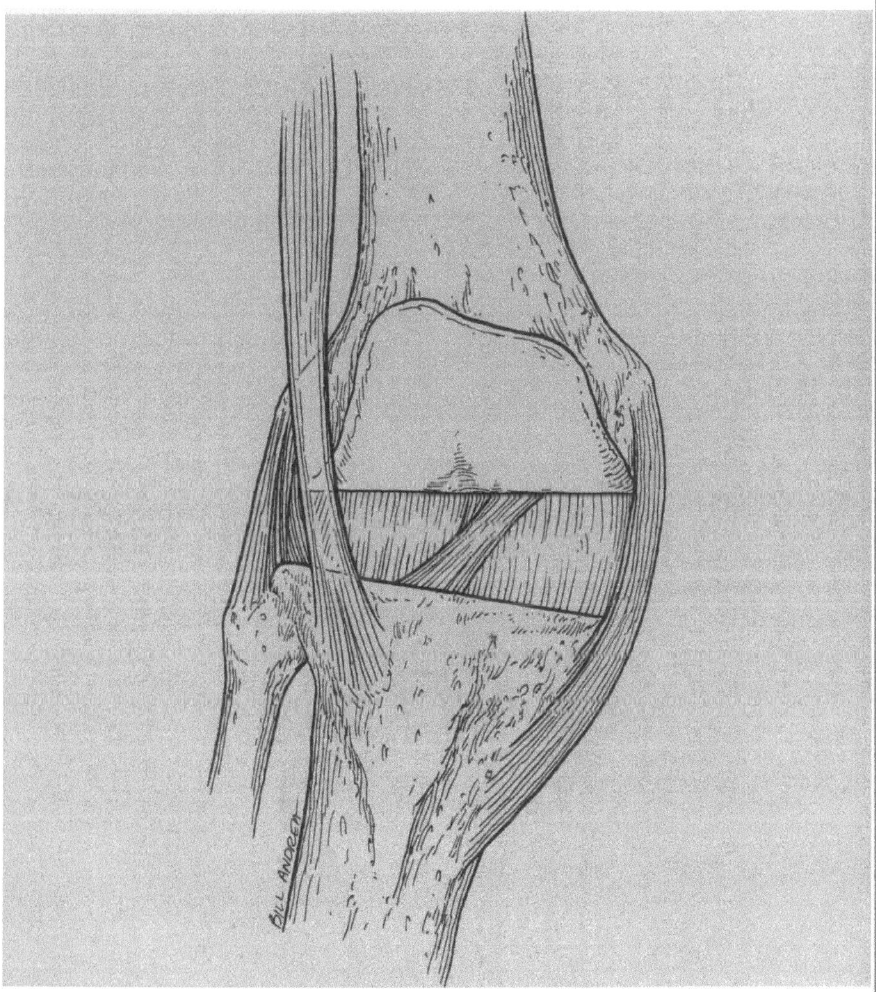

Fig. 145. In this illustration the distal surface of the femur and upper tibia have been resected, and the knee is evaluated for ligament contracture. The knee has lateral contracture in extension, possibly caused by all or just one or two of the lateral structures.

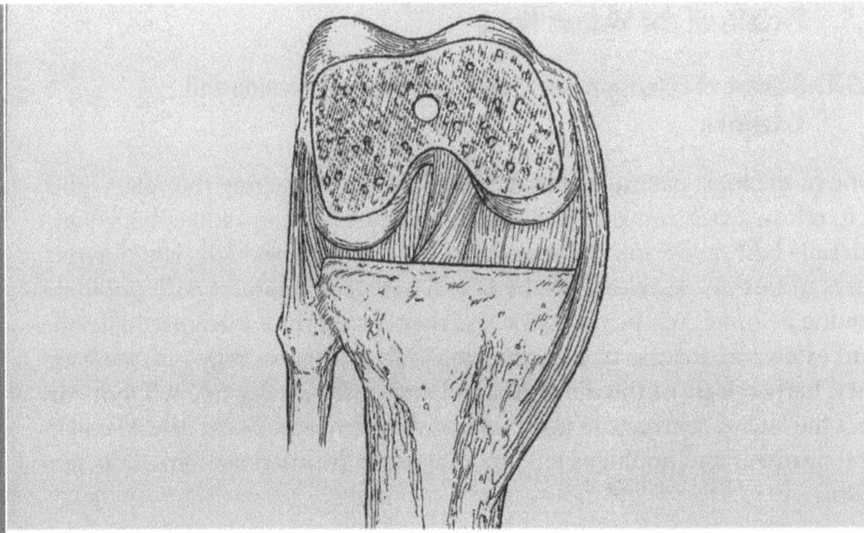

Fig. 146. There also is lateral contracture in flexion. This contracture can only be caused by the lateral collateral ligament, popliteus tendon, or rarely the posterolateral corner, and cannot be caused by the iliotibial band or posterior capsule. It is important to realize that the extension contracture also may be due to the lateral collateral ligament, popliteus tendon, or posterolateral corner, and in many cases, is not caused by the iliotibial band or posterior capsule.

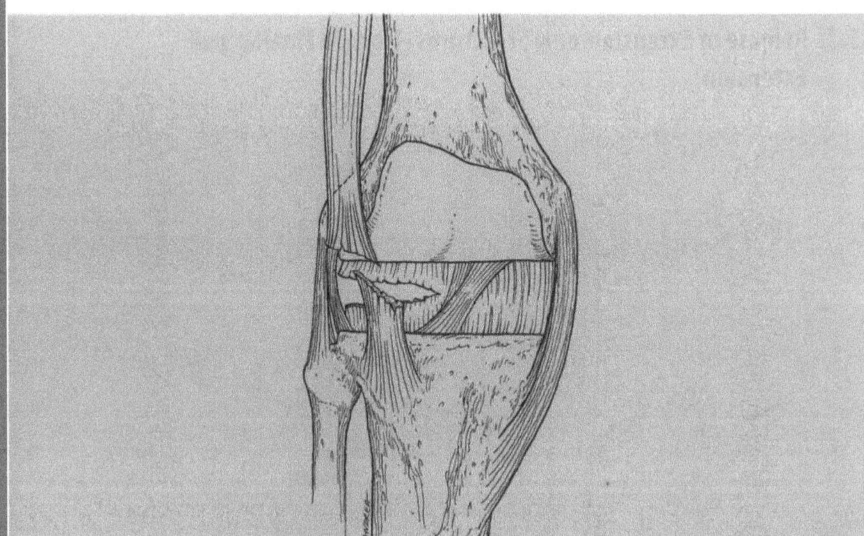

Fig. 147. Release of the iliotibial band and lateral posterior capsule before any of the other ligaments may improve the knee in extension.

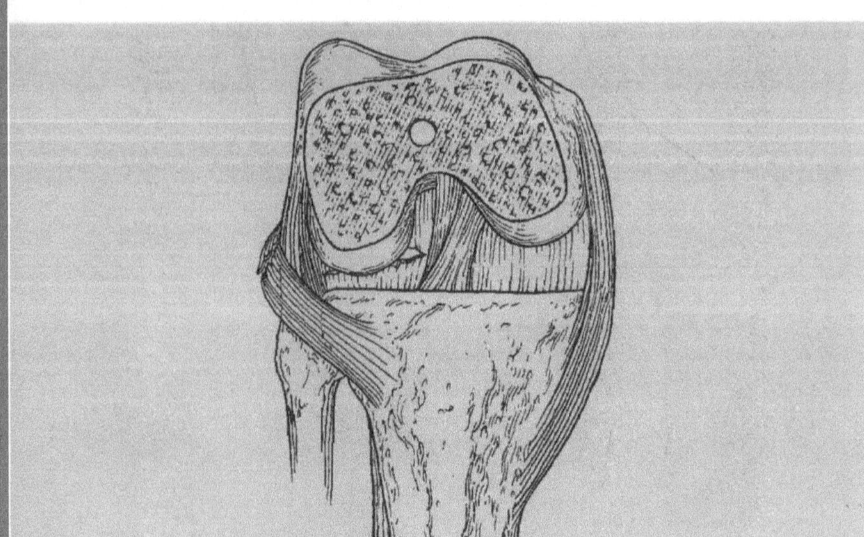

Fig. 148. However, release of the iliotibial band and posterior capsule does not correct the lateral contracture in flexion because only the lateral collateral ligament, popliteus tendon, posterior cruciate ligament, and to a much lesser extent the posterior cruciate ligament, function in flexion.

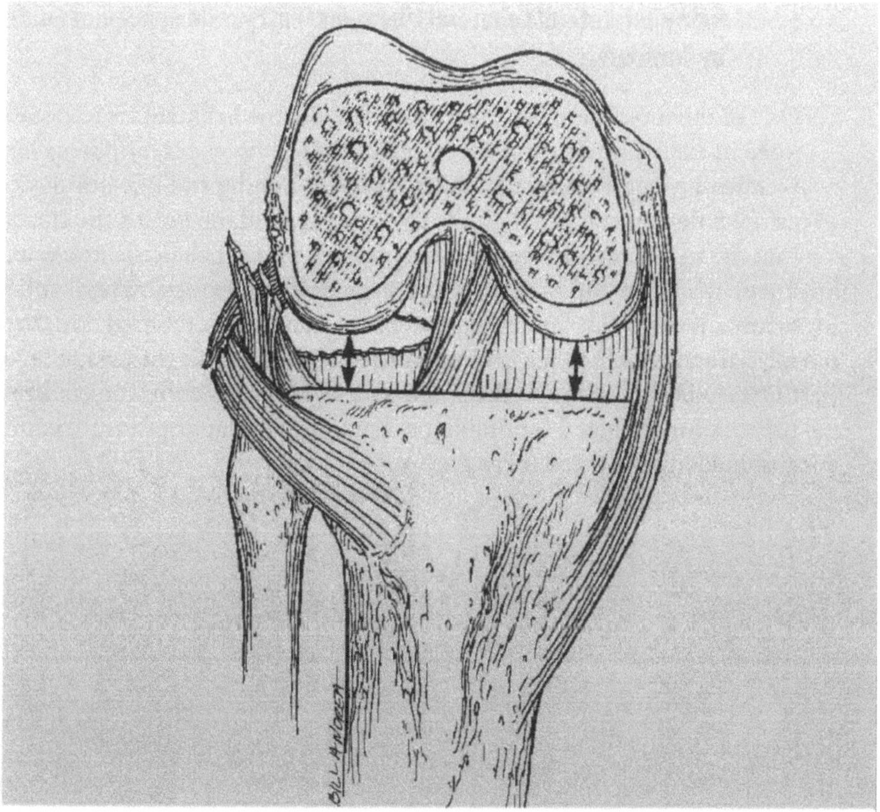

Fig. 149. To correct the lateral contracture in the flexed position, the lateral collateral ligament, popliteus tendon, posterior cruciate ligament, or all three, must be released.

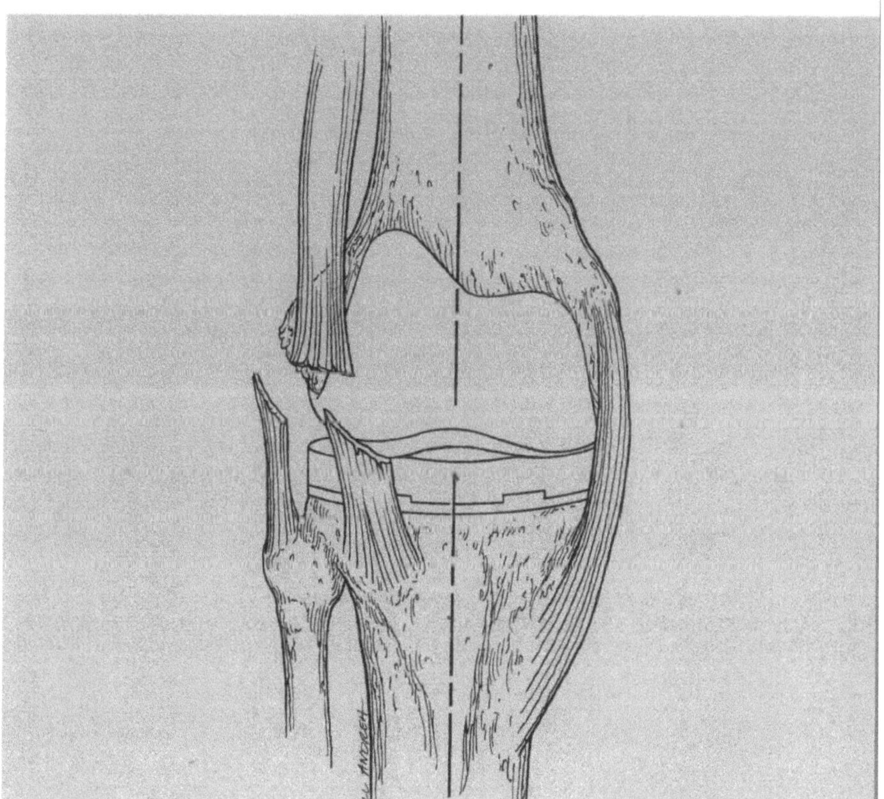

Fig. 150. Now because of the initial release of the iliotibial band and posterior capsule, the knee is excessively lax laterally in extension. This situation can be avoided in knees that are tight laterally both in flexion and extension by releasing the structures first that function both in flexion and extension. This leaves the extension-only structures to provide the vital lateral stability needed for full extension.

5.5.3. Retaining Lateral Collateral Ligament -Cutting Flexion Space Guided by Tensioners

One of the most common errors in balancing the ligaments is to release the knee in extension, leaving the lateral collateral ligament, popliteus tendon or lateral posterior capsule intact, then tensioning the knee in flexion to create a flexion space. When the knee is extended, release of the structures that are tight only in extension may correct the imbalance in the extended knee, but when the knee is flexed the popliteus tendon, lateral collateral ligament, and posterior lateral corner may be considerably tighter than the medial structures. When tensioners are used to distract the joint, the femur is externally rotated, and the flexion surfaces of the femur are cut in internal rotation (valgus), thus failing to correct the valgus deformity in flexion and medializing the patellar groove.

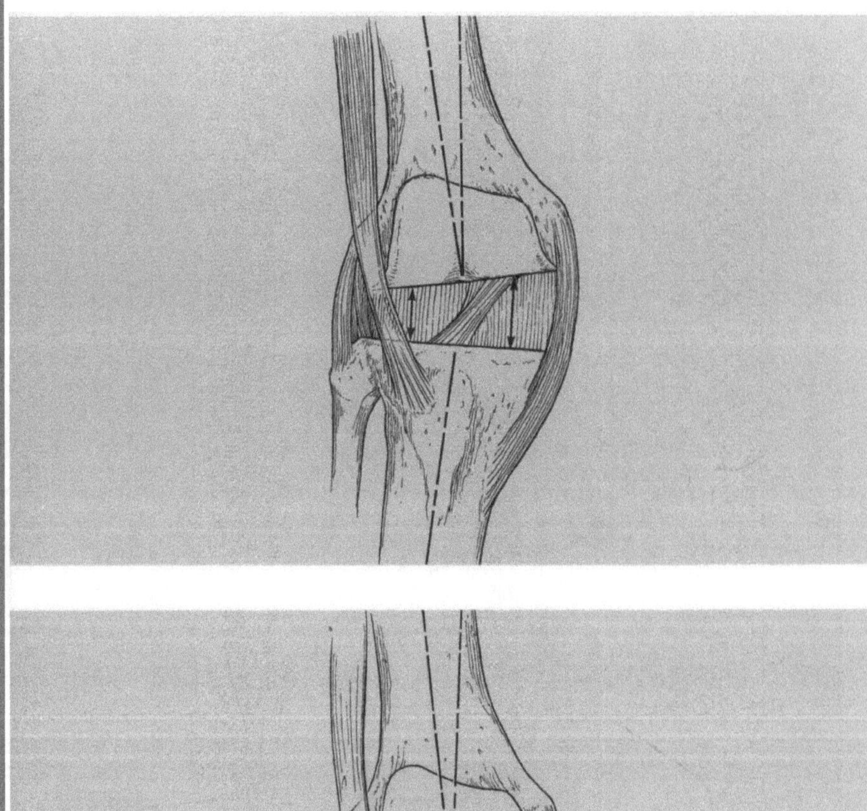

Fig. 151. This knee is tight in extension due to multiple tight lateral structures.

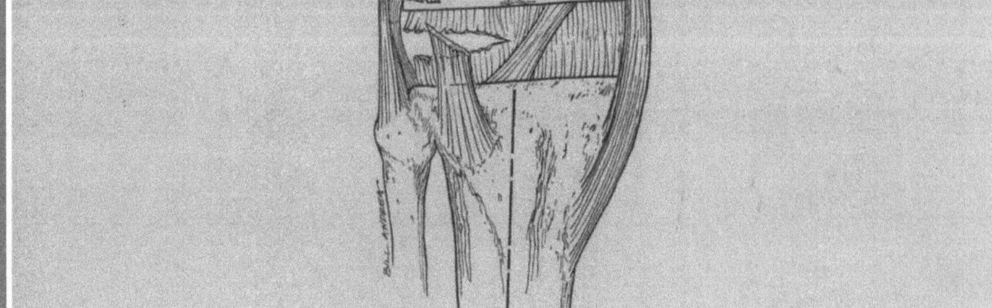

Fig. 152. Release of the iliotibial band and lateral posterior capsule partially corrects the imbalance in extension.

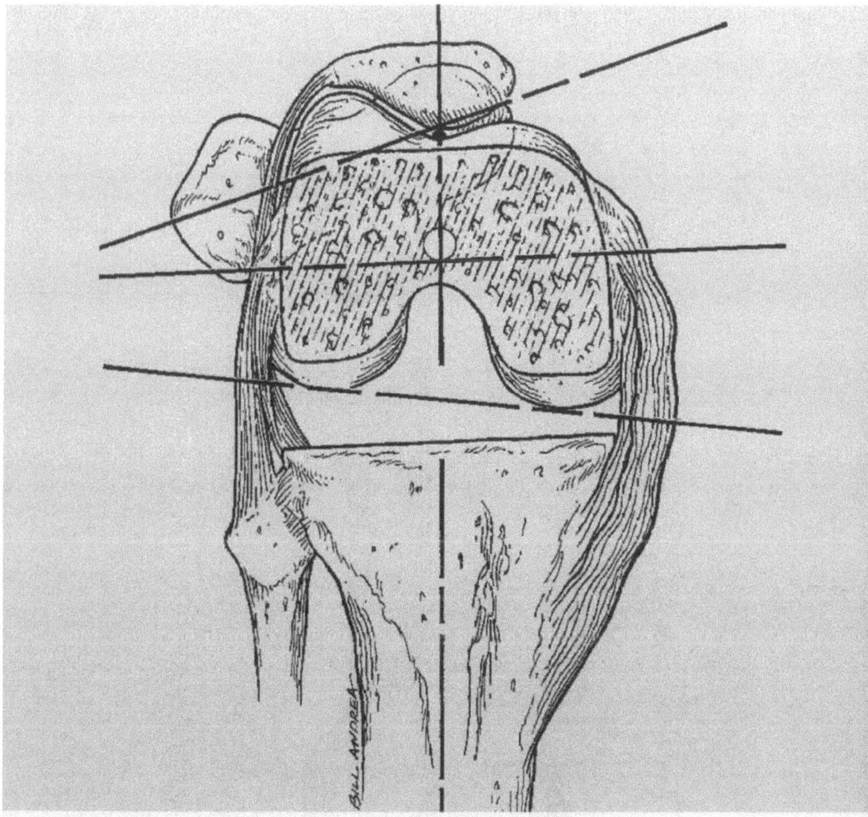

Fig. 153. When the knee is flexed, severe ligament imbalance is not apparent because the lateral femoral condyle is deficient, and thus the lateral collateral ligament and popliteus tendon do not appear to be tight.

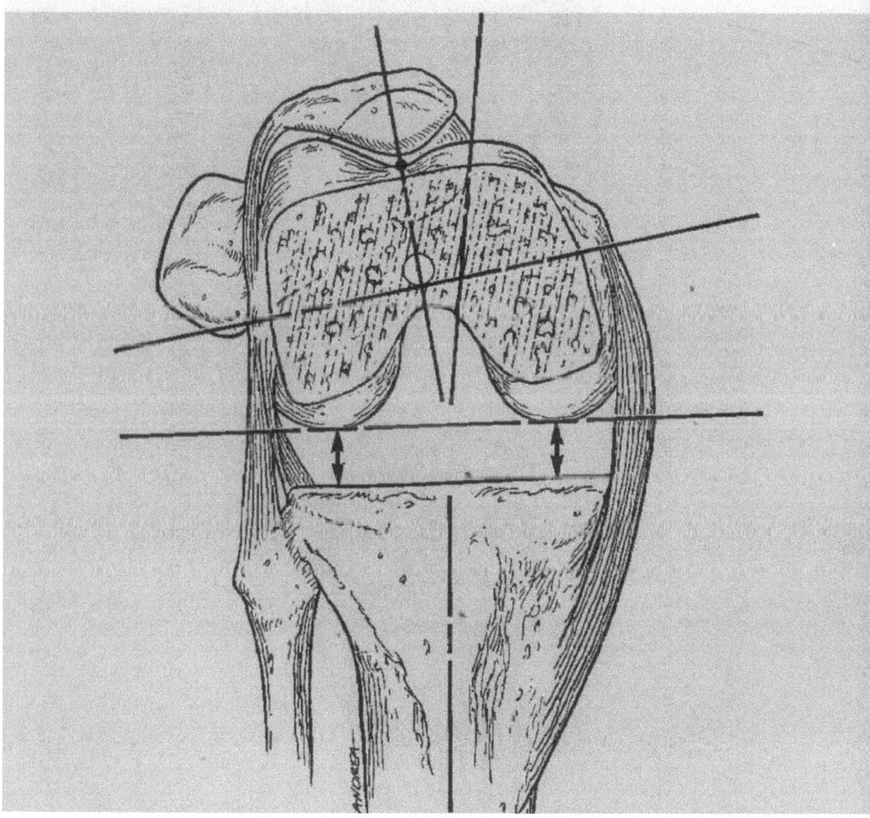

Fig. 154. When tensioners are placed in the joint, the femur rotates externally to tension the loose medial collateral ligament. The joint space may look symmetrical because the lateral femoral condyle is deficient, but the anterior-posterior and epicondylar axes are tilted laterally. The line perpendicular to the joint surface is outside the anterior-posterior plane, and does not point toward the center of the femoral head. The bone cuts are made now, with the femoral and tibial surfaces parallel.

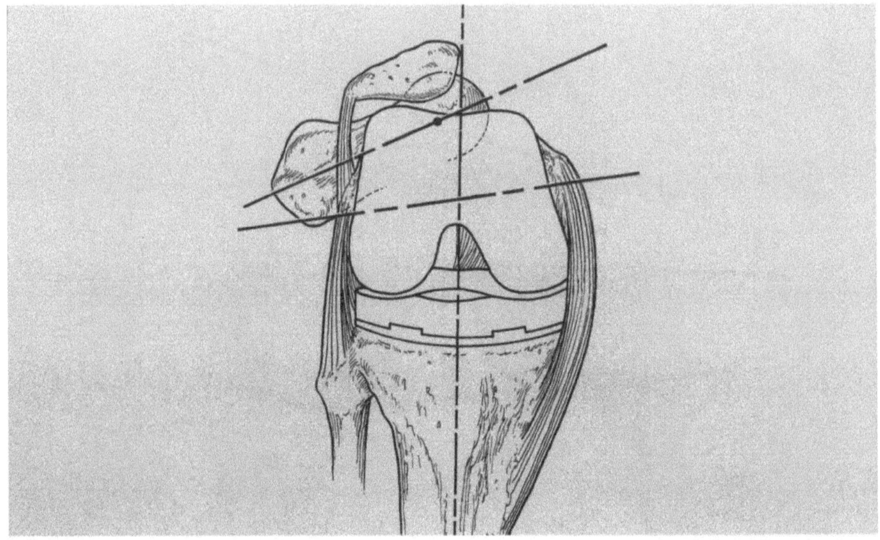

Fig. 155. The components have been inserted with the femur externally rotated and the femoral implants in the new, internally-rotated position. Although the ligaments are balanced, the joint is out of alignment with the femur and the anterior-posterior plane. With the tibia held vertically, the hip is externally rotated and the epicondylar axis is tilted externally. The patella is positioned laterally relative to the new patellar groove. The patellar groove does not point toward the center of the femoral head.

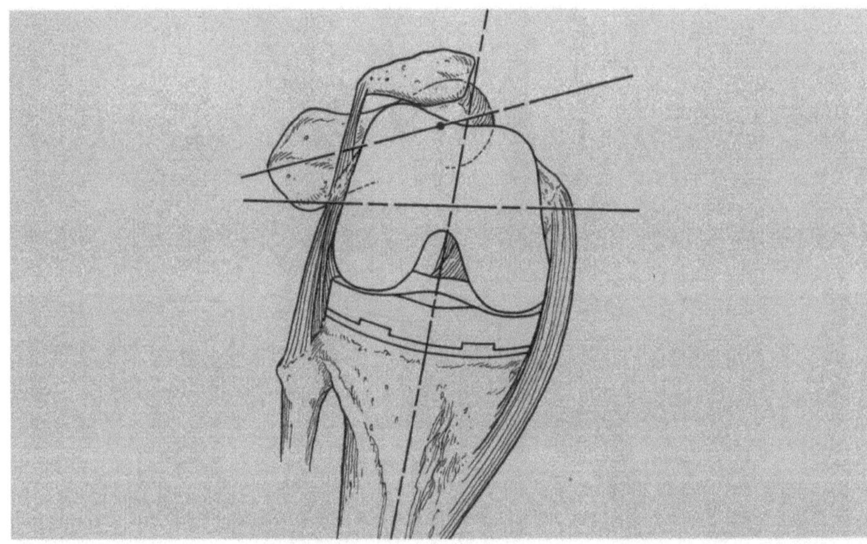

Fig. 156. When the hip is allowed to return to its functional position, and the epicondyles are parallel to the floor, the tibia assumes a valgus position, and it is apparent that the femoral component is internally rotated. The patella is positioned laterally relative to the new patellar groove. The patellar groove does not point toward the center of the femoral head.

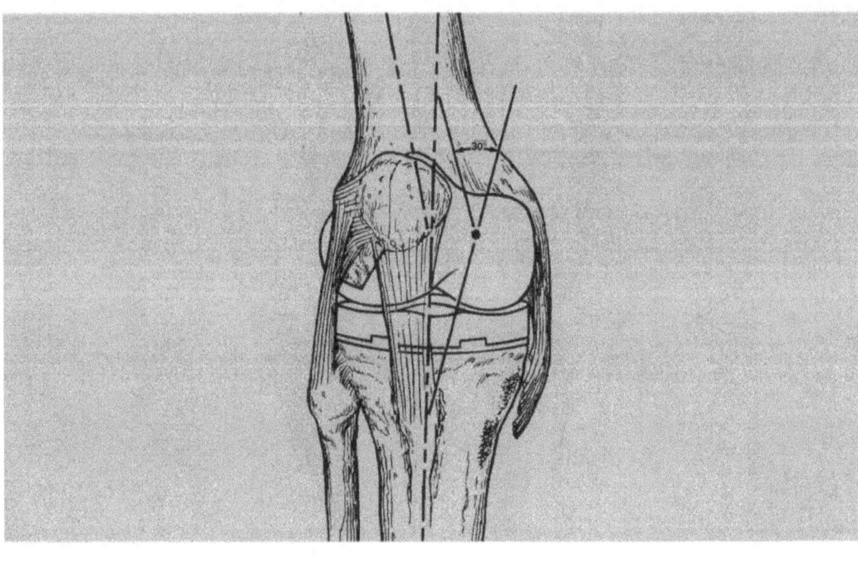

Fig. 157. With the knee fully extended, varus-valgus alignment is close to normal because the long axes of the femur and tibia were used to establish alignment in extension. However, the internally rotated femoral component places the patellar groove medially, and lateral patellar subluxation occurs because of the excessive Q-angle (approximately 30°).

5.5.4. Using the Deficient Lateral Condyle as Reference for Bone Resection

In knees with severe lateral femoral condylar deficit, one of the common pitfalls is to overresect the distal femur to achieve bone resection of the distal surface of the lateral femoral condyle. This raises the joint in extension, making flexion-extension balancing difficult, and the medial bone resection may encroach on the bone attachment of the medial collateral ligament.

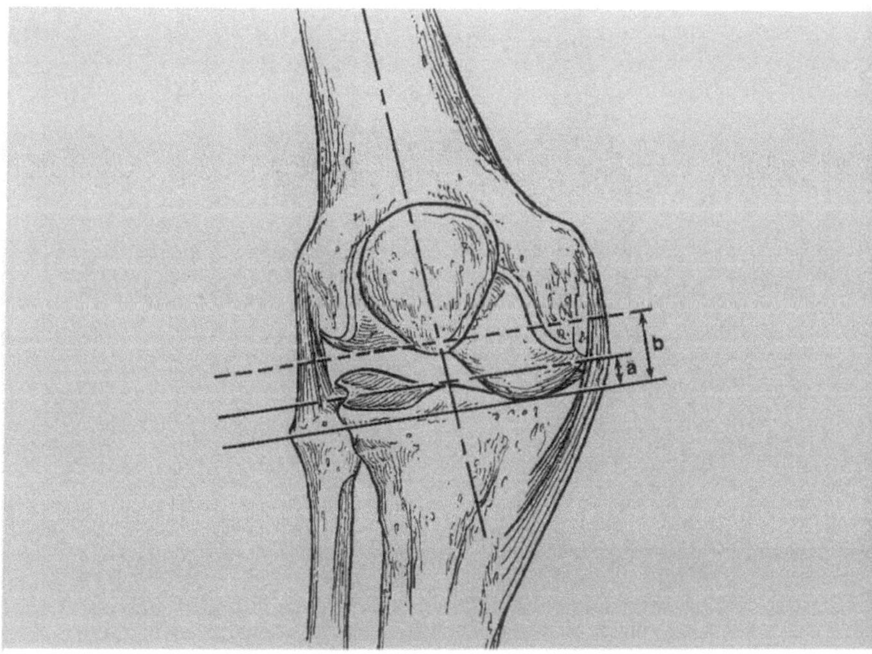

Fig. 158. In this illustration the distance b represents the amount of distal femoral resection necessary to achieve contact with bone on the distal lateral side of the knee, and distance a is the thickness of the femoral implant. Overresection to the level indicated raises the joint level in extension, and the resection may even encroach on the femoral attachment of the medial collateral ligament.

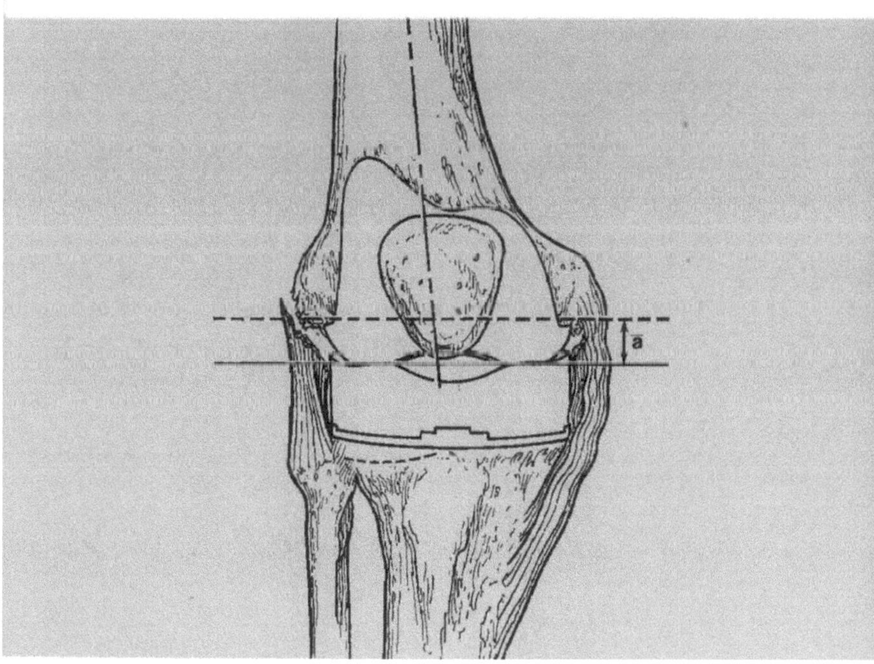

Fig. 159. The thickness of the femoral implant (a) is inadequate to tension the medial collateral ligament, so a much thicker tibial polyethylene component is used. The lateral ligaments have been released to correct abnormal lateral tightness, but the medial ligaments may be so loose that they may require advancement or even substitution with a stabilized implant. The joint line has been raised, so that patellar impingement is likely in flexion.

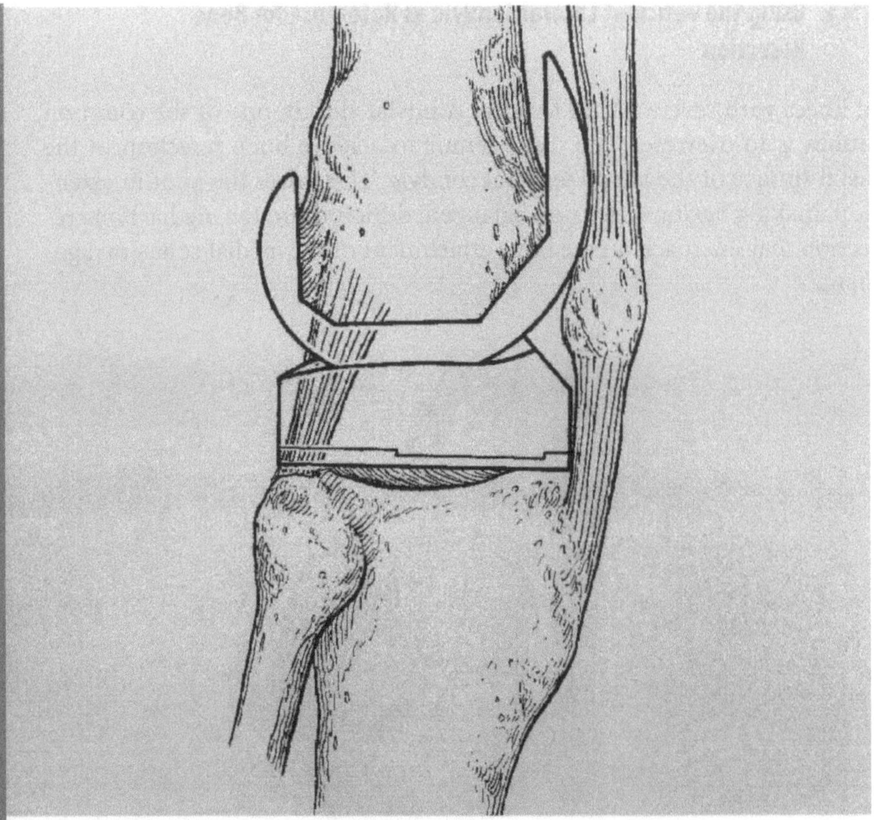

Fig. 160. Problems caused by the elevated joint involve the posterior cruciate ligament and patella. Unless the posterior femoral surface is overresected to an extent equal to that of the distal medial surface, the thicker tibial component used to stabilize the knee in extension will cause the knee to be too tight in flexion. Here the posterior cruciate ligament is at normal tension in extension because the overresection of the femur is matched by the thickness of the tibial component. The tibial component impinges anteriorly against the inferior pole of the patella as the knee flexes. In full extension the impingement is not apparent.

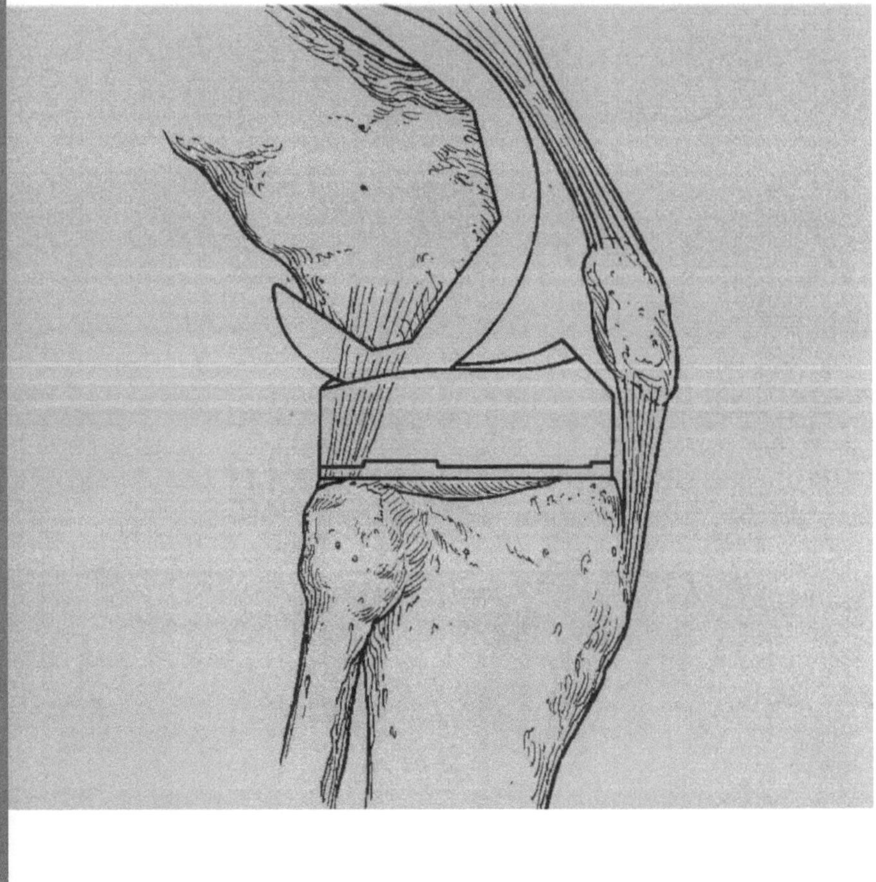

Fig. 161. As the knee flexes, the thick tibial polyethylene component causes the knee to be too tight, and the posterior cruciate ligament enforces excessive rollback of the femoral component also the collateral ligaments are likely to be too tight in flexion. The patella impinges against the anterior edge of the tibial component.

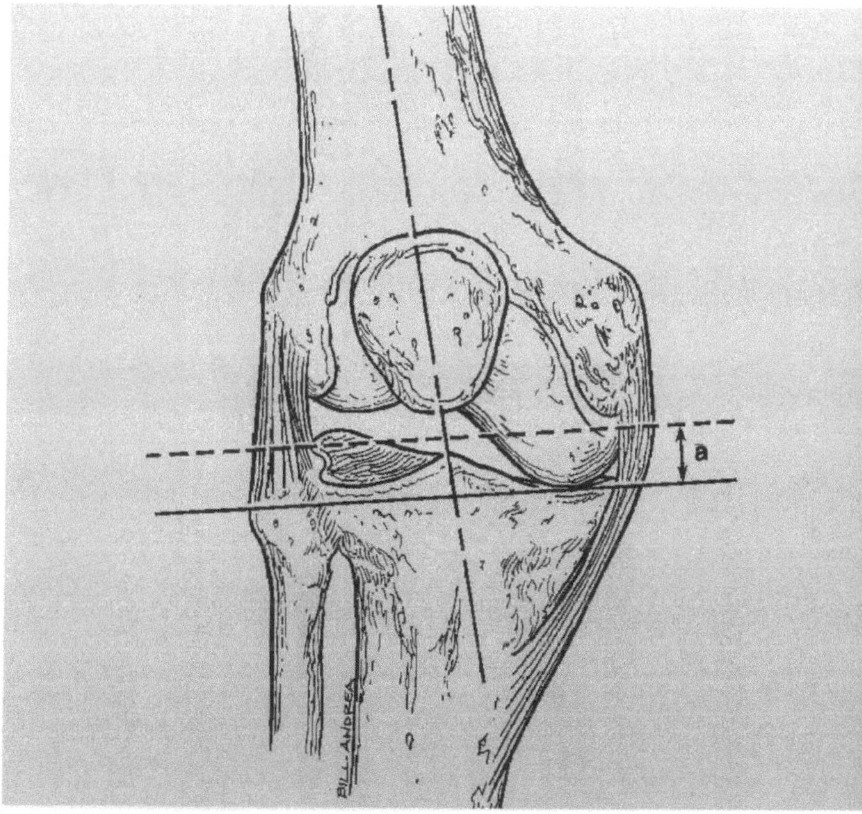

Fig. 162. The solution to this problem is to use the intact medial side as the point of reference for resection, positioning the cutting guide to resect the thickness of the implant (a). In cases with severe lateral deficiency, this position of resection will remove nothing from the distal surface of the lateral femoral condyle. However, the anterior and posterior bevel surfaces of the femur will almost always be resected, creating a surface on which to rest the femoral component.

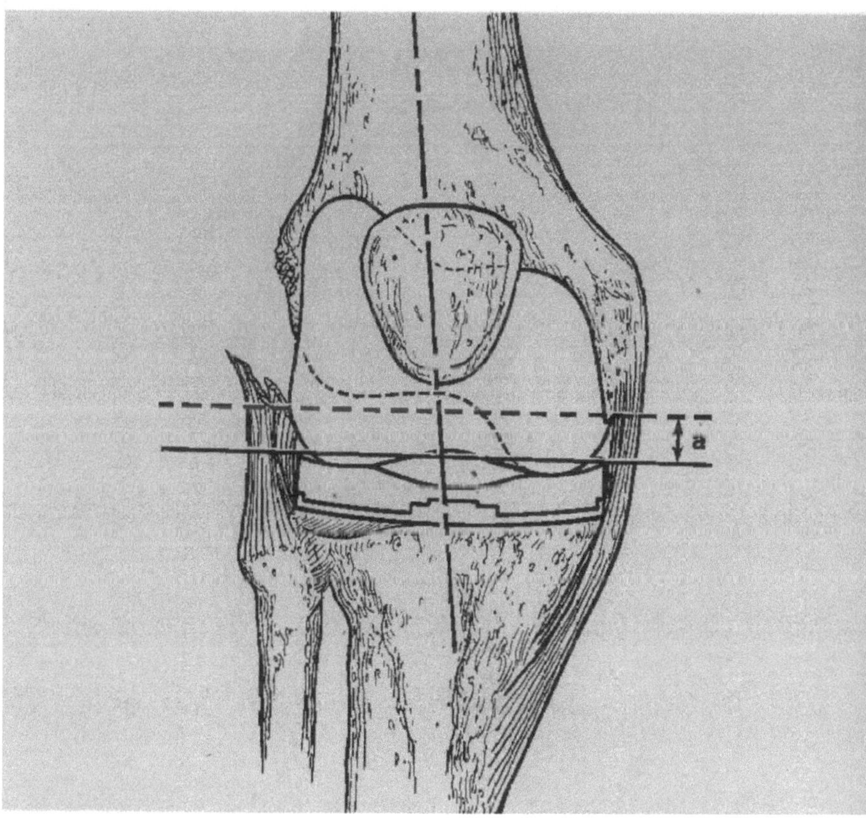

Fig. 163. With the femoral surface resected at the proper level by resecting the thickness of the component (a) from the medial joint surface, the medial collateral ligament is easier to tension correctly, and the extremely thick tibial component is not necessary. Lateral ligament releases are done as necessary to accommodate the added structure in the lateral side of the knee.

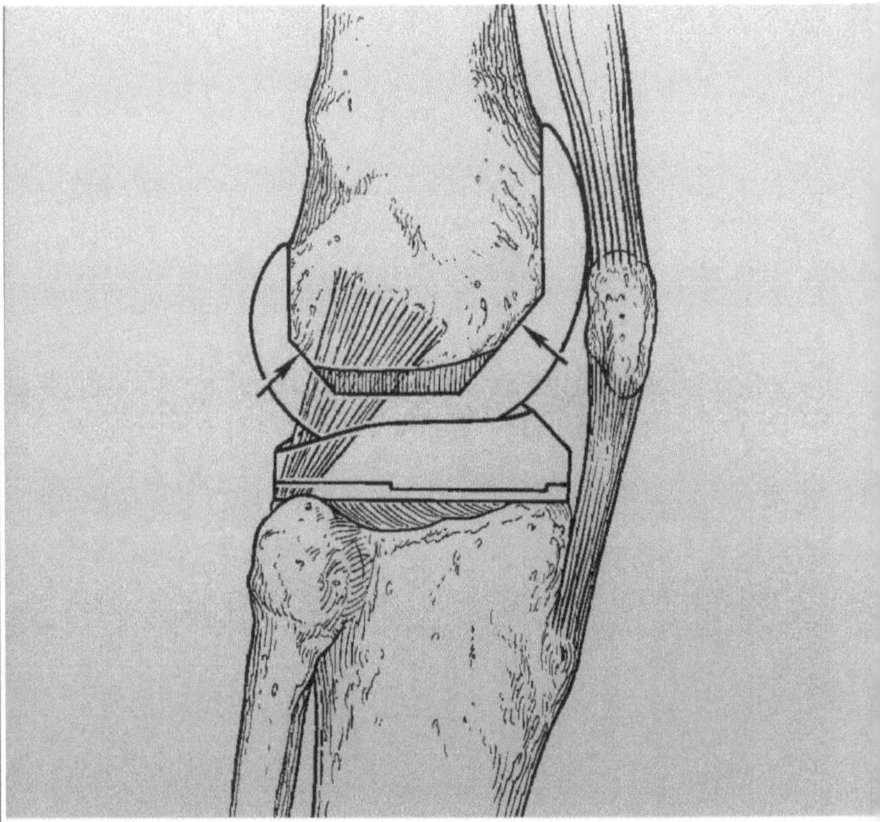

Fig. 164. Although the distal surface of the femur is not resected and does not support the implant, the anterior bevel surface has been resected, and provides all the lateral support necessary to stabilize the femoral component. The patella and posterior cruciate ligament now are positioned appropriately in flexion and extension.

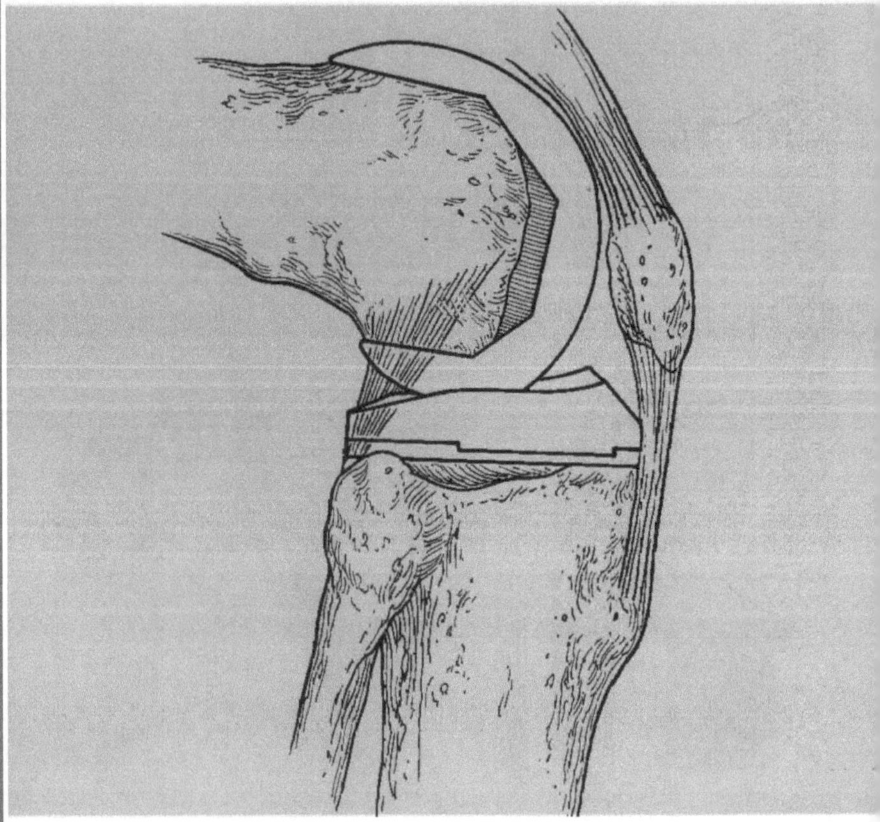

Fig. 165. When the knee flexes the posterior cruciate ligament and patella function normally, allowing normal positioning of the femoral surface on the tibial surface.

Suggested Readings

1. Anouchi YS, Whiteside LA, Kaiser AD, Milliano MT: The effect of axial rotational alignment of the femoral component on knee stability and patellar tracking in total knee arthroplasty. Clin Orthop 287:170–177, 1991.
2. Arima J, Whiteside LA, White SE, McCarthy DS. Femoral rotational alignment in the valgus total knee arthroplasty based on the anterior-posterior axis: a technical note. J Bone Joint Surg 77A:1331–1334, 1995.
3. Basmajian JV, Lovejoy JF: Functions of the popliteus muscle in man. J Bone Joint Surg Am 53:557–562, 1971.
4. Burks RT: Gross anatomy. In Daniel D, Akeson W, O'Connor J (eds). Knee Ligaments: Structure, Function, Injury, and Repair. New York, Raven Press 59–76, 1990.
5. Crowninshield R, Pope MH, Johnson RJ: An analytical model of the knee. J Biomech 9:397–405, 1976.
6. Gollehon DL, Torzilli PA< Warren RF: The role of the posterolateral and cruciate ligaments in the stability of the human knee. J Bone Joint Surg Am 69:233–242, 1987.
7. Goodfellow J, O'Connor J. Mechanics of the knee and prosthesis design. J Bone Joint Surg 60B:358–369, 1978.
8. Grood ES, Noyes FR, Butler DJ, Suntay WJ: Ligamentous and capsular restraints preventing straight medial and lateral laxity in intact human cadaver knees. J Bone Joint Surg 63A:1257–1269, 1981.
9. Grood ES, Stowers SF, Noyes FR: Limits of movement in the human knee. J Bone Joint Surg 70A:88–97, 1988.
10. Hull ML, Berns GS, Varma H, Patterson HA: Strain in the medial collateral ligament of the human knee under single and combined loads. J Biomech 29:199–206, 1996.
11. Hsieh HH, Walker PS: Stabilizing mechanisms of the loaded and unloaded knee joint. J Bone Joint Surg Am 58:87–93, 1976.
12. Insall J, Ranawat CS, Scott WN, Walker P. Total condylar knee replacement. Preliminary report. Clin Orthop 120:149–154, 1976.
13. Markolf KL, Mensch JS, Amstutz HC: Stiffness and laxity of the knee-the contributions of the supporting structures. J Bone Joint Surg Am 58:583–594, 1976.
14. Martin JW, Whiteside LA: The influence of joint line position on knee stability after condylar knee arthroplasty. Clin Orthop 259:146–156, 1990.
15. Trent PS, Walker PS, Wolf B. Ligament length patterns, strength, and rotational axes of the knee joint. Clin Orthop 117:263–270, 1976.
16. Whiteside LA: Intramedullary alignment of total knee replacement. A clinical and laboratory study. Orthop Review (suppl) 9–12, 1989.
17. Whiteside LA: Correction of ligament and bone defects in total arthroplasty of the severely valgus knee. Clin Orthop 288:234–245, 1993.
18. Whiteside LA, Arima J: The anterior-posterior axis for femoral rotational alignment in valgus total knee arthroplasty. Clin Orthop 321:168–172, 1995.
19. Whiteside LA, Kasselt MR, Haynes DW: Varus and valgus and rotational stability in rotationally unconstrained total knee arthroplasty. Clin Orthop 219:147–157, 1987.
20. Whiteside LA, McCarthy DS: Laboratory evaluation of alignment and kinematics in a unicompartmental knee arthroplasty inserted with intramedullary instrumentation. Clin Orthop 274:238–247, 1992.
21. Whiteside LA, Summers RG: Anatomical landmarks for an intramedullary alignment system for total knee replacement. Orthop Trans 7:546–547, 1983.
22. Whiteside LA, Summers RG: The effect of the level of distal femoral resection on ligament balance in total knee replacement. In Dorr LD (ed). The Knee: Papers of the First Scientific Meeting of the Knee Society. Baltimore, University Park Press 59–73, 1984.
23. Yoshioka Y, Siu D, Cooke TDV: The anatomy and functional axes of the femur. J Bone Joint Surg 69A:873–880, 1987.

Flexion Contracture and Femoral Sizing

6. Flexion Contracture and Femoral Sizing

Basic Principles

Flexion contracture in most knees is caused by tight collateral ligaments, so major alterations in bone resection should not be done until all ligaments have been balanced to acceptable tension. Specifically, the distal femur should not be overresected until all ligaments are balanced and all osteophytes are resected.

One issue that should be considered early is the effect of femoral size on ligament tightness in flexion and extension. The femoral component should be slightly oversized to tighten the flexion space so that the tibia can be over-resected to loosen the extension space without excessive loosening of the flexion space. The tibial surface is resected perpendicular to the long axis of the tibia in the sagittal plane to resect more anteriorly than posteriorly, thus loosening the extension space.

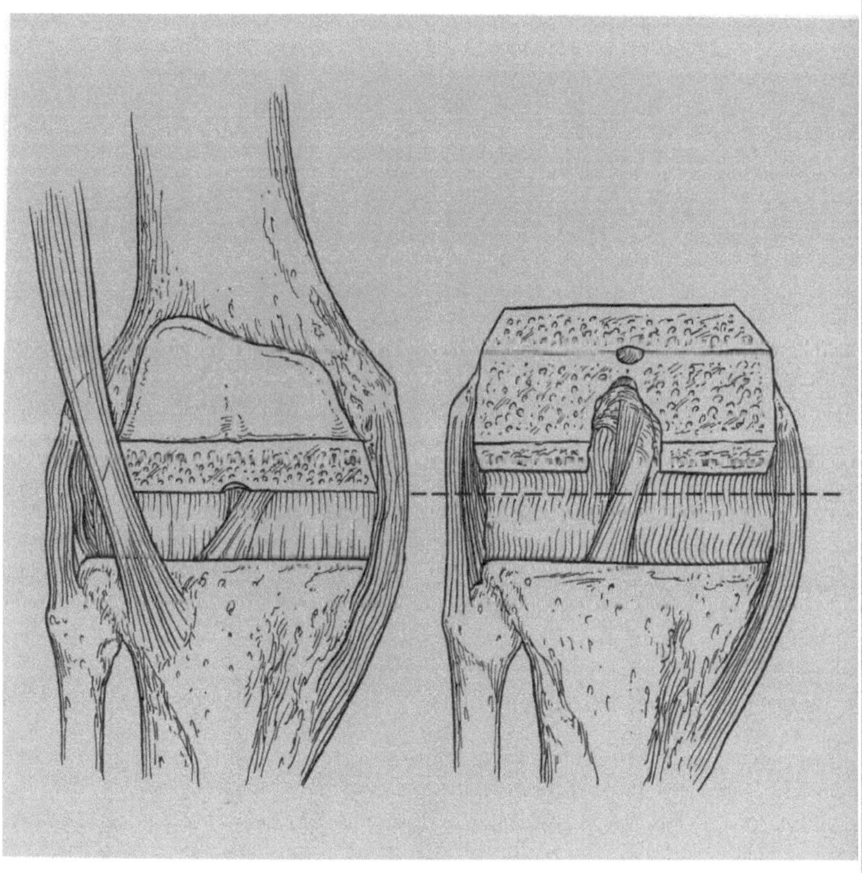

Fig. 166. When dealing with a flexion contracture, it is helpful to consider the flexion gap as being too large and the extension gap as being too small. The ligaments that are effective primarily in extension, the iliotibial band, posterior portion of the medial collateral ligament, and posterior capsule are overly effective. The ligaments that are effective primarily in flexion, the lateral collateral ligament, popliteus complex, and the anterior portion of the medial collateral ligament, are relatively ineffective.

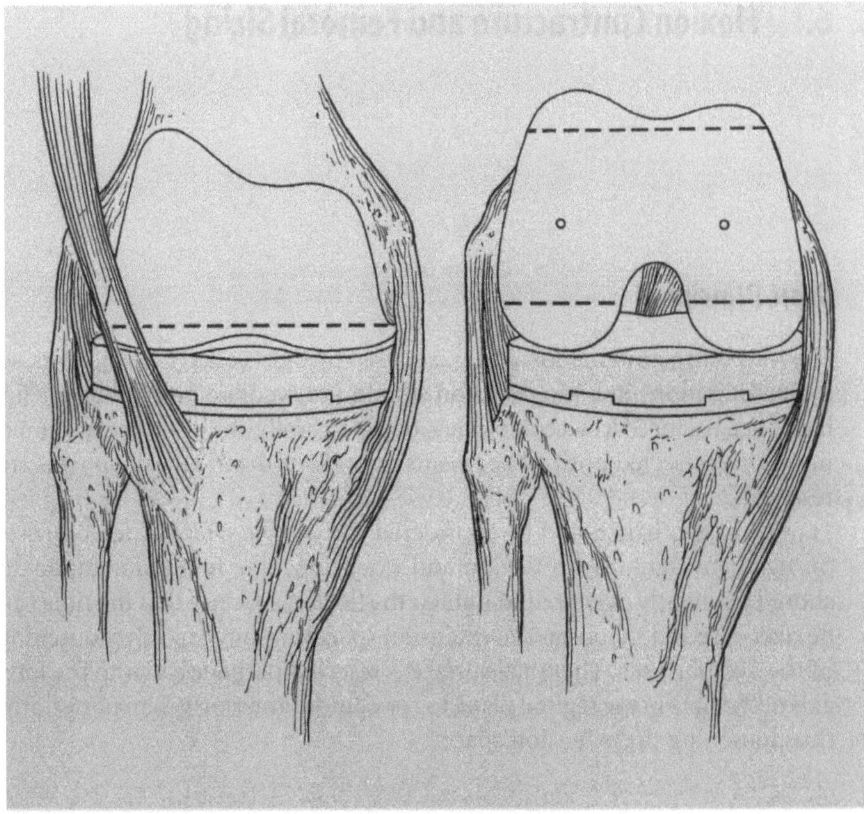

Fig. 167. The larger femoral component does not change the distal surface of the femur or the extension space. As usual, the thickness of the femoral component is removed from the distal surface of the femur. More is resected from the upper surface of the tibia than the thickness of the implant to allow the knee to extend fully. Less than the thickness of the femoral component is resected from the posterior aspect of the femur. This tightens the flexion space, and makes up for the over-resection of the distal tibia that was done to loosen the extension space.

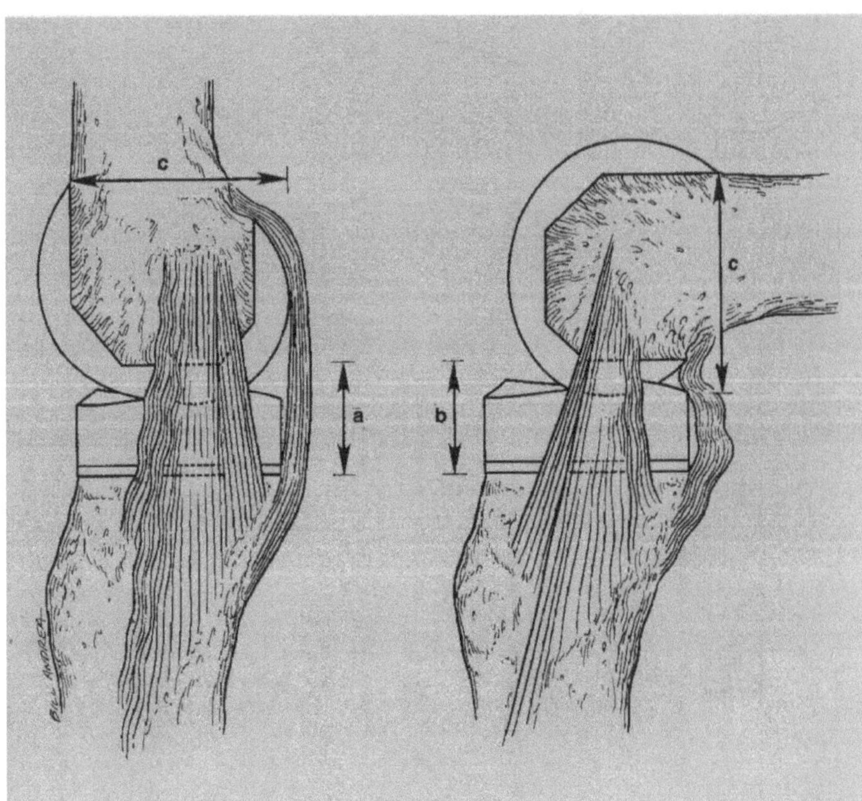

Fig. 168. Viewed from the side, it is clear that a larger femoral component, when placed properly with anterior referencing, resects less posterior bone and lengthens the distance from front-to-back (c). This tightens the flexion (b) space to make it more closely match the extension space (a).
The proximal tibial surface has been resected perpendicular to the long axis of the tibia to remove more bone anteriorly than posteriorly. This increases the extension space and makes knee extension easier.

6.1. Varus Knee with Flexion Contracture

Most flexion contractures are caused by tight collateral ligaments and posterior capsule, and often are worsened by osteophyte impingement under these ligaments. The first step in treating flexion contracture is thorough removal of osteophytes. Then the ligaments should be assessed. Tight ligaments then should be released until the ligaments are properly balanced, and again the flexion contracture should be reassessed. Almost all flexion contracture is alleviated by ligament balancing, leaving very few knees in need of resection of more distal femoral bone.

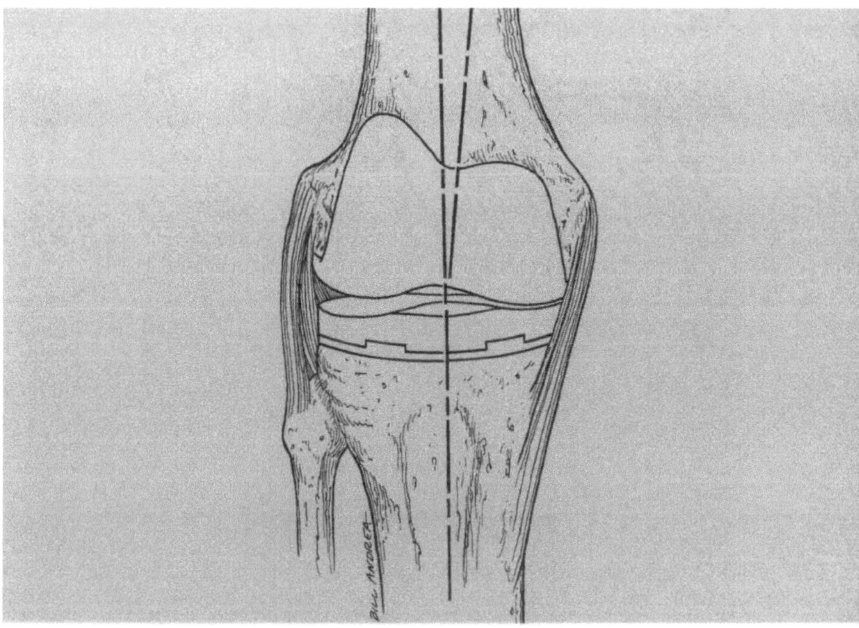

Fig. 169. After insertion of trial implants, this knee still has varus deformity because of tight medial collateral ligaments. The joint surface gapes spontaneously laterally and the knee is very tight medially to valgus stress.

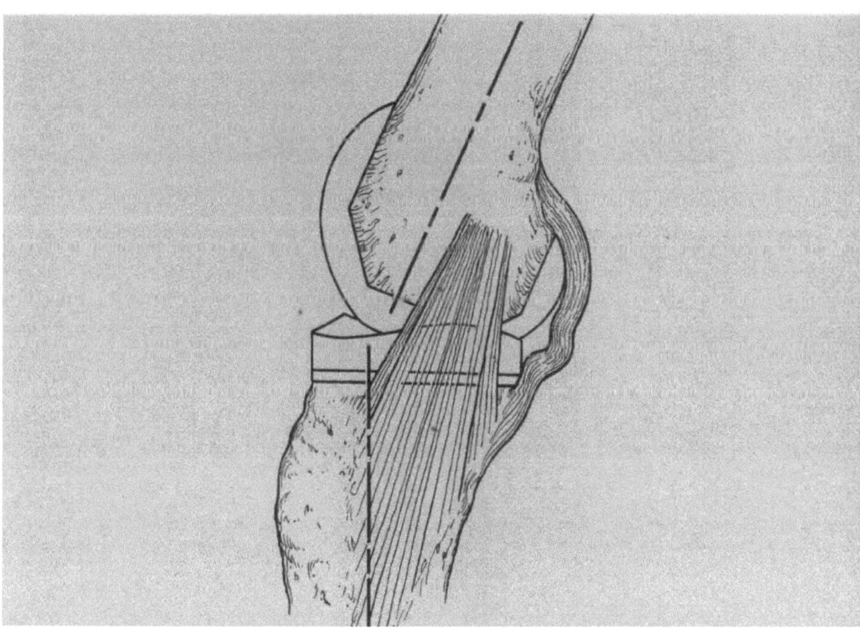

Fig. 170. Extension of the knee is limited by the tight medial collateral ligament, and the posterior capsule is not brought to full tension because of this checkrein effect of the medial collateral ligament.

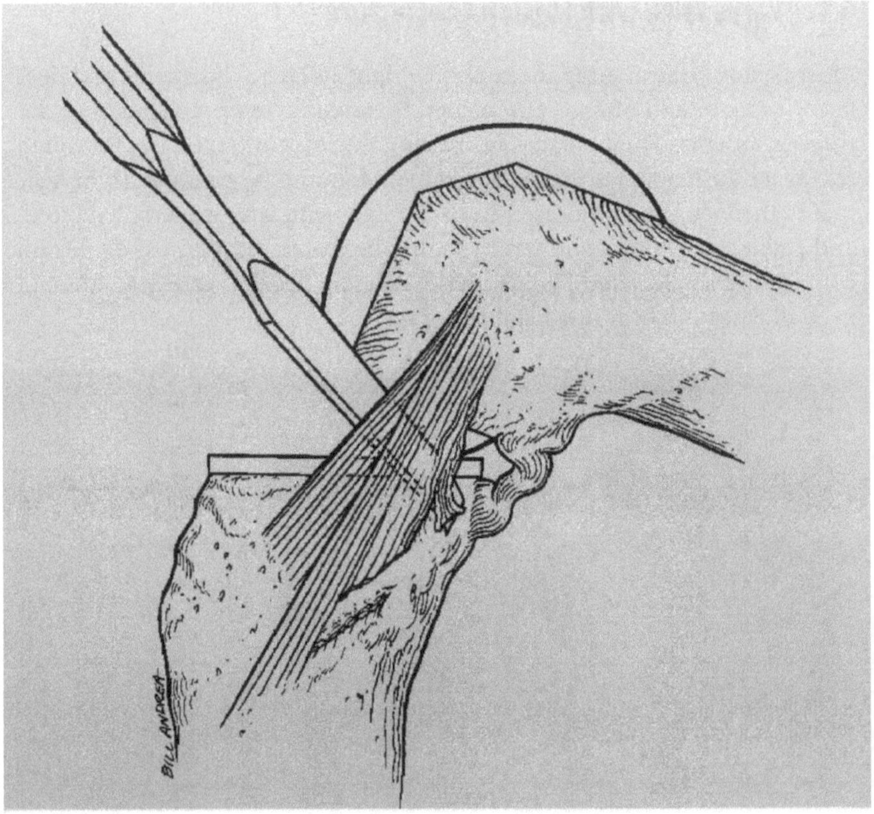

Fig. 171. The sequence of releases is very important in this case. The single structure most likely to cause both the flexion contracture and tight medial structures is the posterior portion of the medial collateral ligament. This is released first, and stability and range of motion are checked again. Most likely the knee will still be tight medially after posterior release of the medial collateral ligament. If the knee is still abnormally tight medially and still has a flexion contracture, the anterior portion of the medial collateral ligament is released.

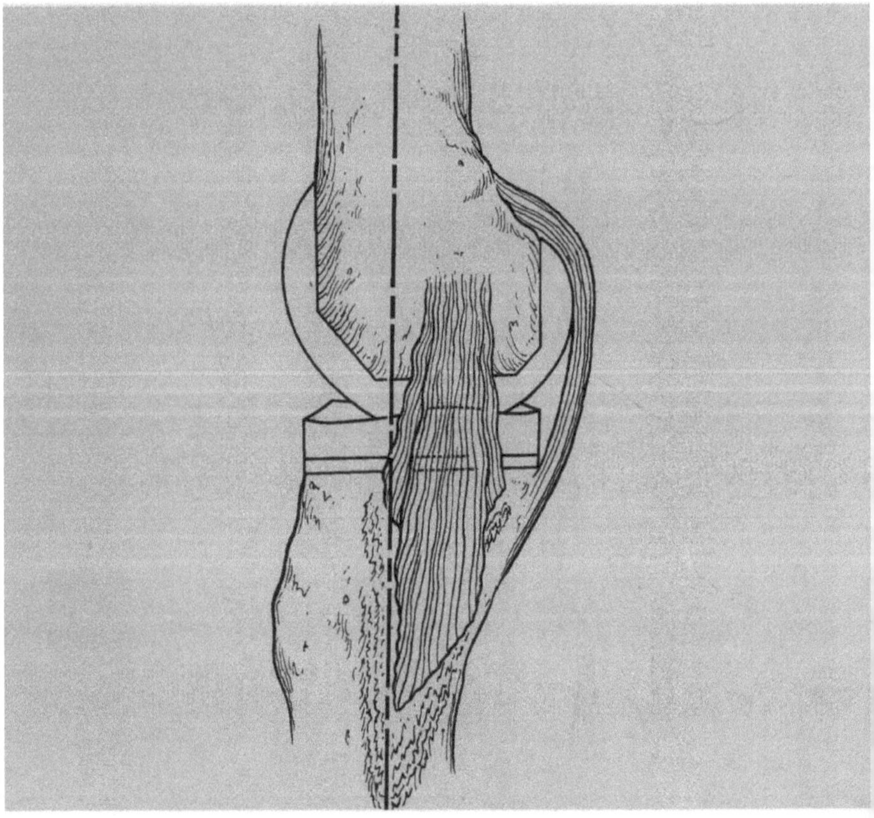

Fig. 172. Now the medial collateral ligament has been released completely, and the flexion contracture has been corrected. The posterior capsule is tensioned normally with the knee in full extension, and acts as a secondary medial stabilizer in extension. Caution: the posterior capsule should not be released first when there is medial collateral ligament tightness combined with flexion contracture. The flexion contracture probably is caused by the medial collateral ligament, and release of the posterior capsule would not correct the flexion contracture. Then when the medial collateral ligament finally is released, the knee will be too loose medially in extension.

Occasionally after complete balance of the knee has been achieved in flexion and extension, the knee still will not extend because of persistent tightness in the posterior capsule.

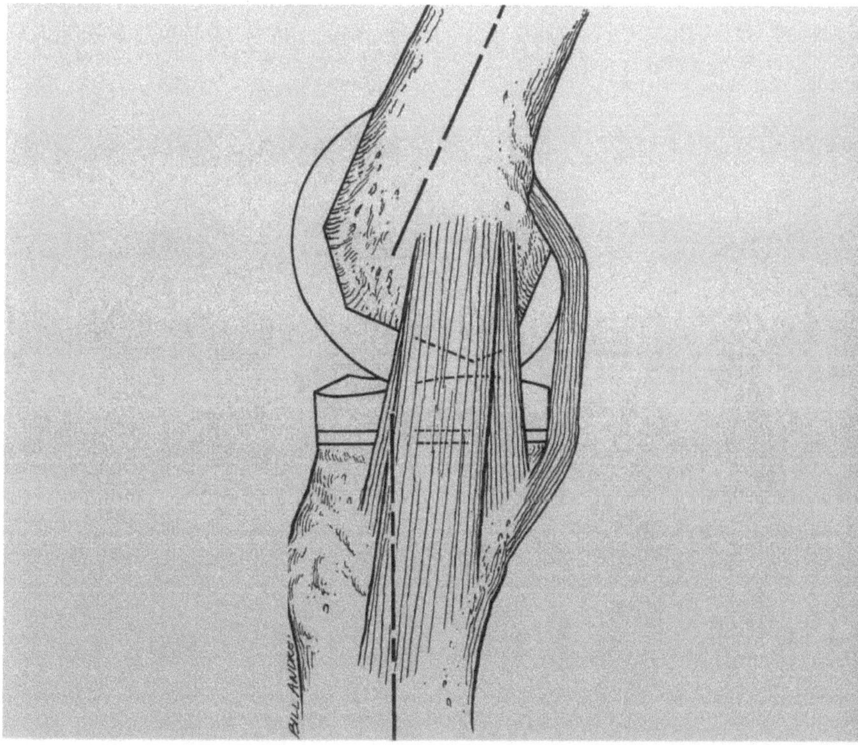

Fig. 173. In the case illustrated, medial and lateral stability are normal, but the knee will not extend. The posterior capsule is tight, but the collateral ligaments are not.

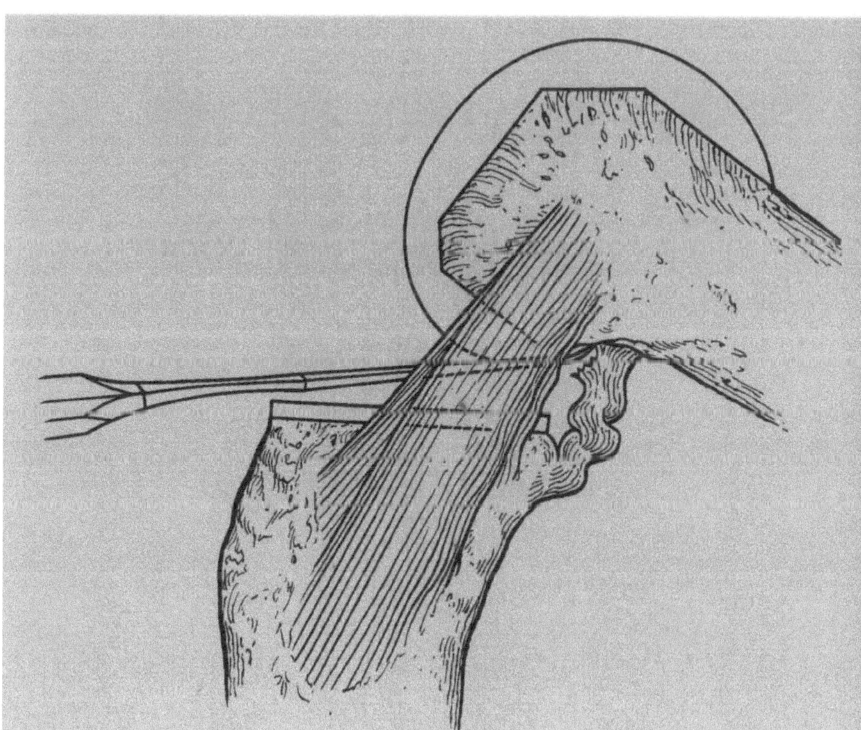

Fig. 174. The tibial trial polyethylene components have been removed, and a curved 1/2-inch osteotome is used to elevate the posterior capsule from its femoral attachment.

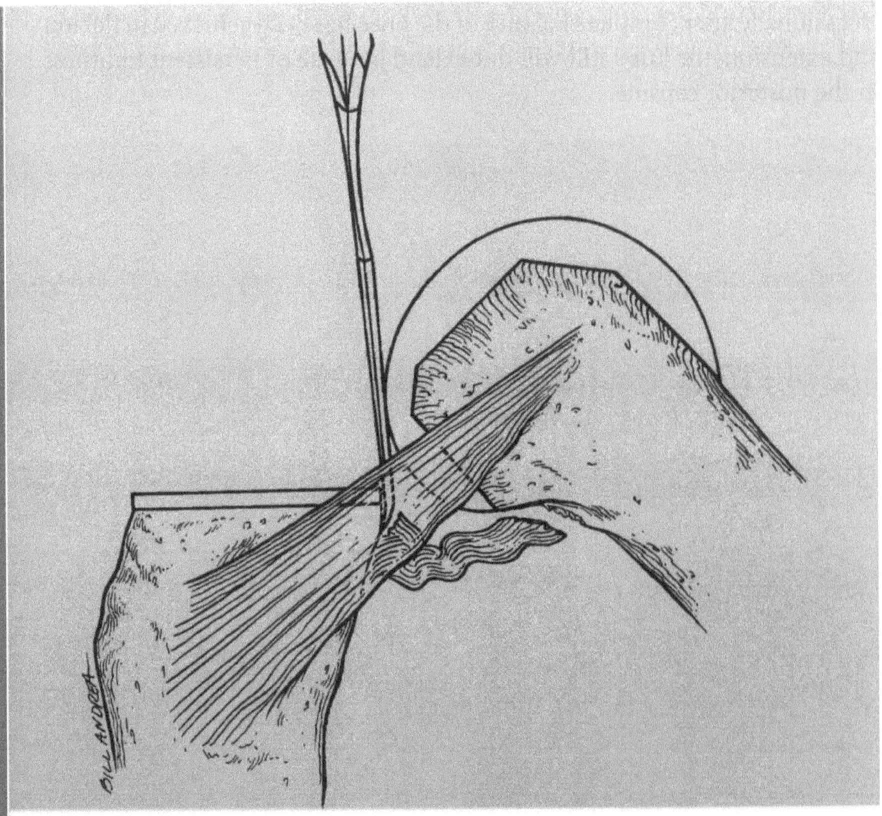

Fig. 175. With the knee in hyperflexion, the posterior-medial capsule also is elevated from its tibial attachment. It is unsafe to detach the posterior capsule from the lateral tibial surface because the peroneal nerve is easily damaged with this procedure.

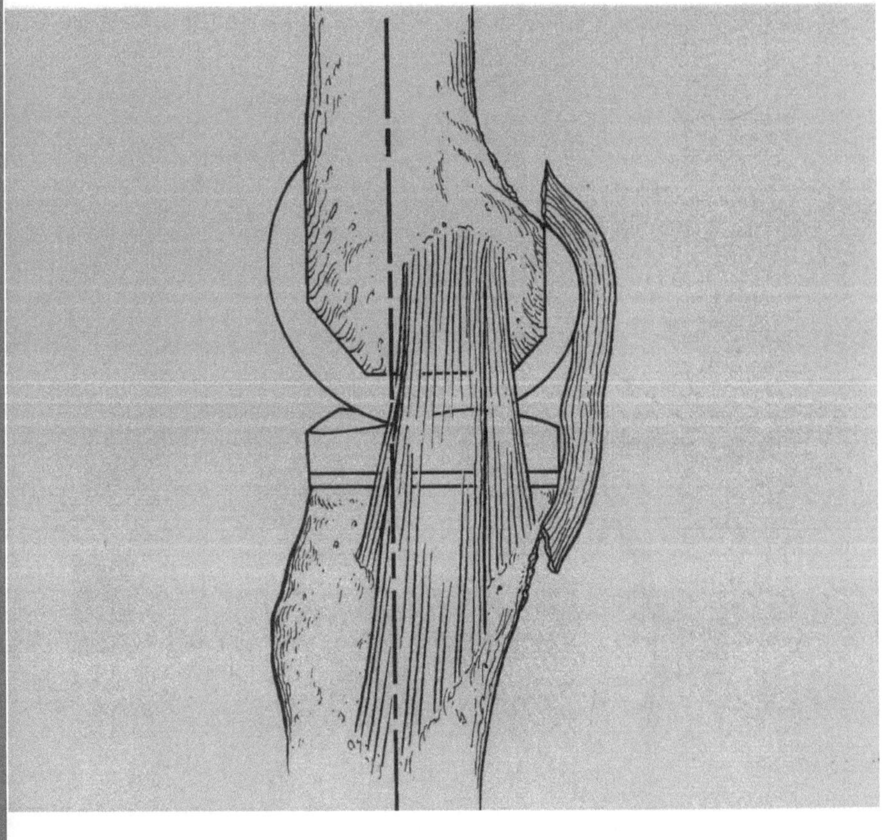

Fig. 176. Now the knee extends fully, and the collateral ligaments are tensioned normally.

Only rarely does flexion contracture persist after correction of collateral ligament imbalance and release of the posterior capsule. In these few cases, more bone should be resected distally from the femur to loosen the knee in extension.

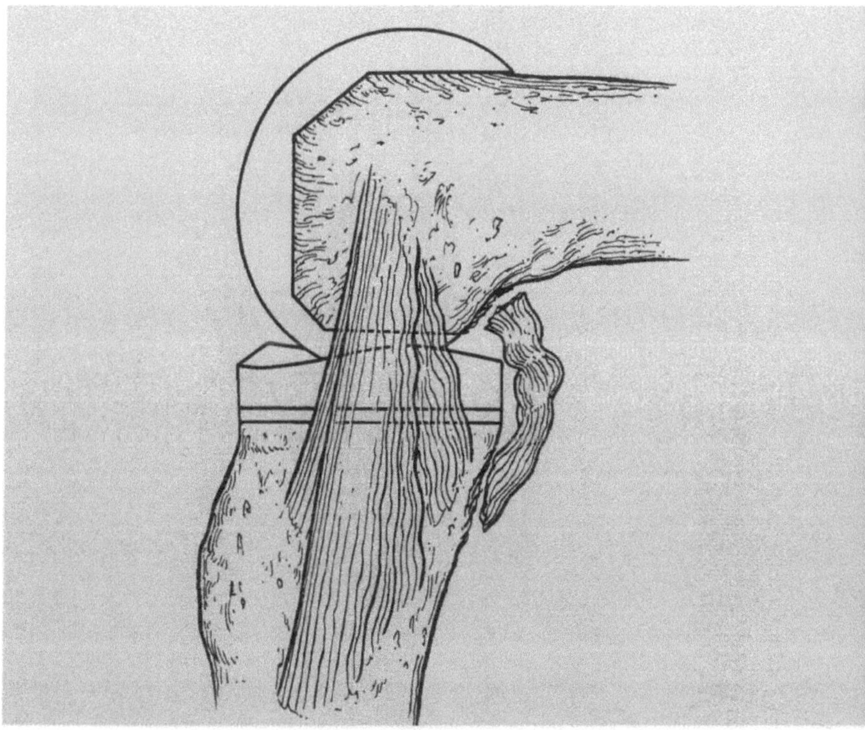

Fig. 177. The knee is well balanced in flexion. The collateral ligaments are tensioned appropriately, and the femoral surface sits correctly on the surface of the tibial component.

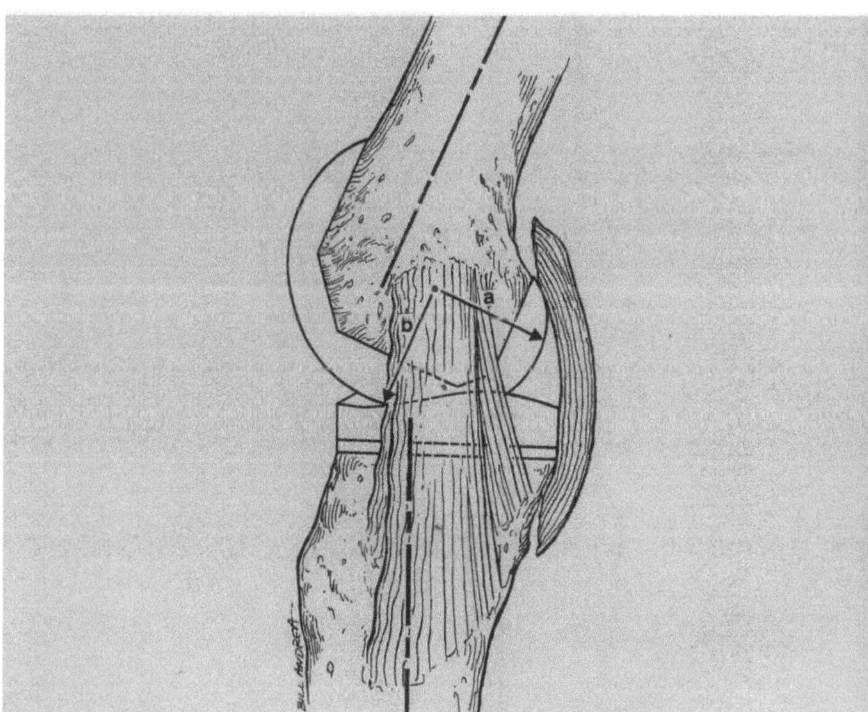

Fig. 178. In extension both the medial and lateral collateral ligaments are too tight to allow full extension. Because stability is acceptable in flexion, distance (a) should stay the same, but distance (b) must be shortened to allow the knee to extend fully.

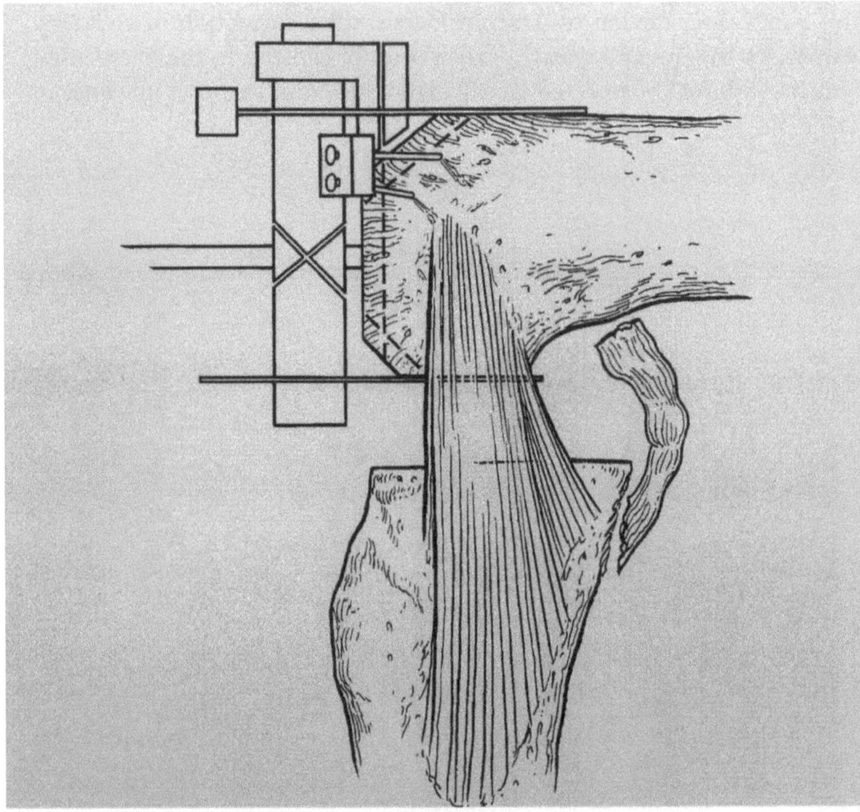

Fig. 179. Distal resection is done to decrease the cam effect of the femur in extension. Shims are used to position the resection guide to not resect anterior or posterior bone, and the guide is placed to resect about 5 mm from the distal surface of the femur.

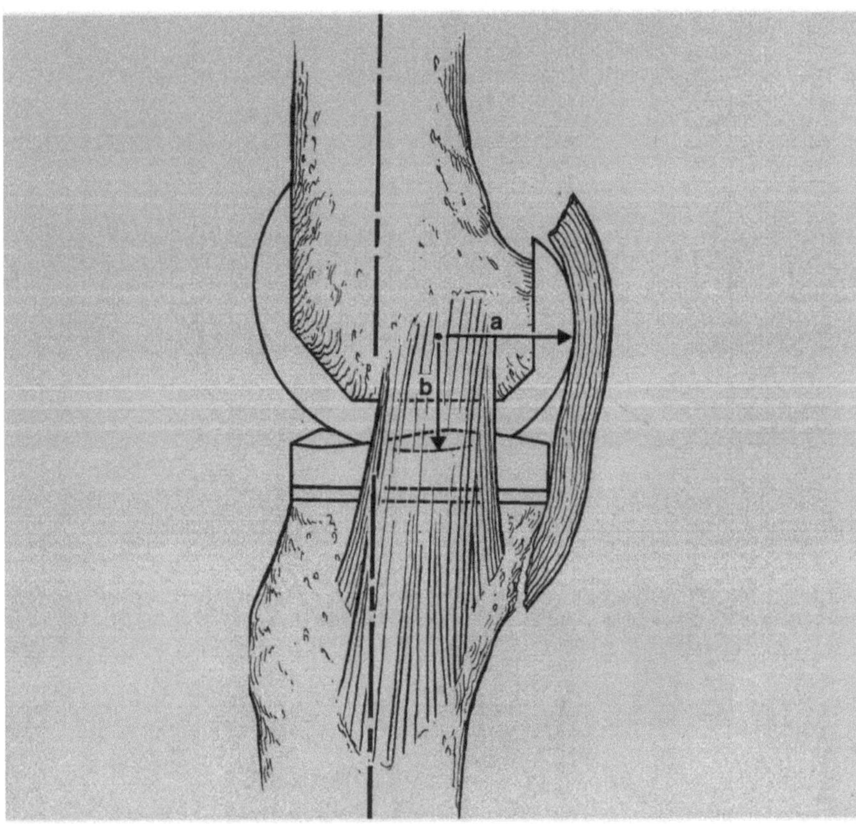

Fig. 180. Distance "b" has been shortened, so that the knee extends completely, and medial-lateral stability is maintained. Because distance a has not been changed, knee stability is unchanged in flexion.

6.2. Pitfalls with Flexion Contracture

Overresection of the distal femur to correct flexion contracture before ligament balancing and osteophyte excision

One of the most common pitfalls encountered in dealing with the knee with flexion contracture is ignoring the effect of ligament contracture and osteophytes on extension of the knee. Although early overresection of the distal femur may straighten the knee, it leads to serious imbalance between flexion and extension once the osteophytes are removed and the knee is balanced.

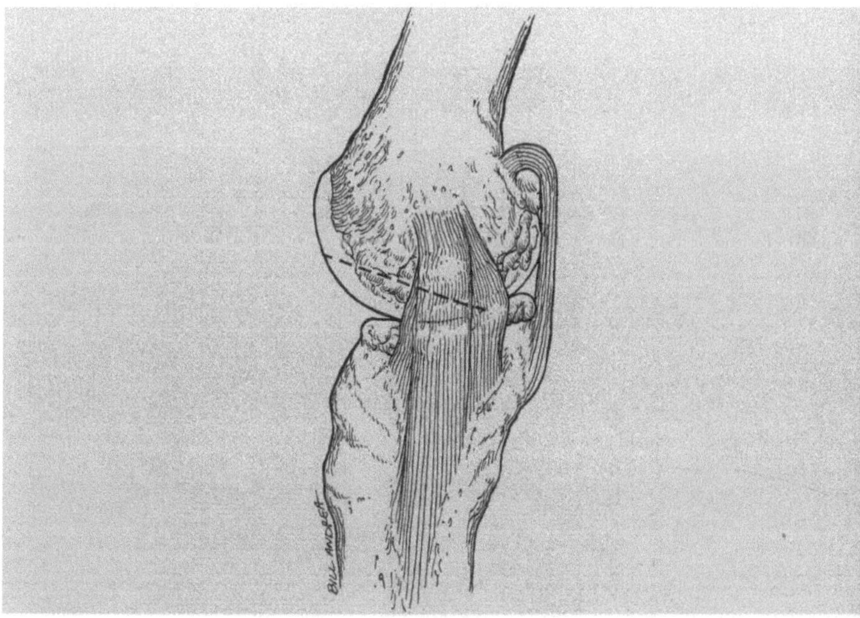

Fig. 181. The knee will not extend fully, but is restrained by tight medial collateral ligaments and joint line osteophytes that tent the ligaments and tension the posterior capsule.

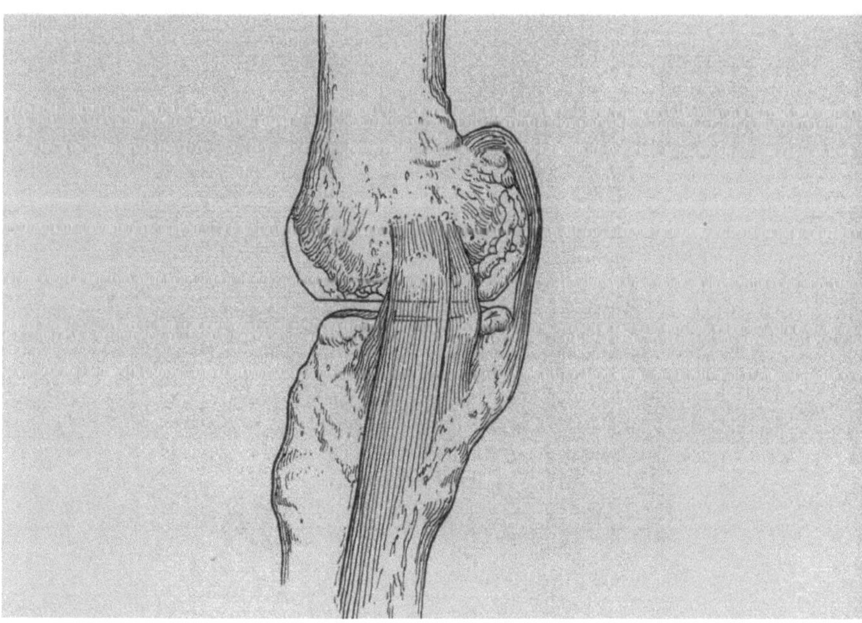

Fig. 182. The distal surface of the femur has been resected to achieve full extension before removal of osteophytes and balancing of ligaments.

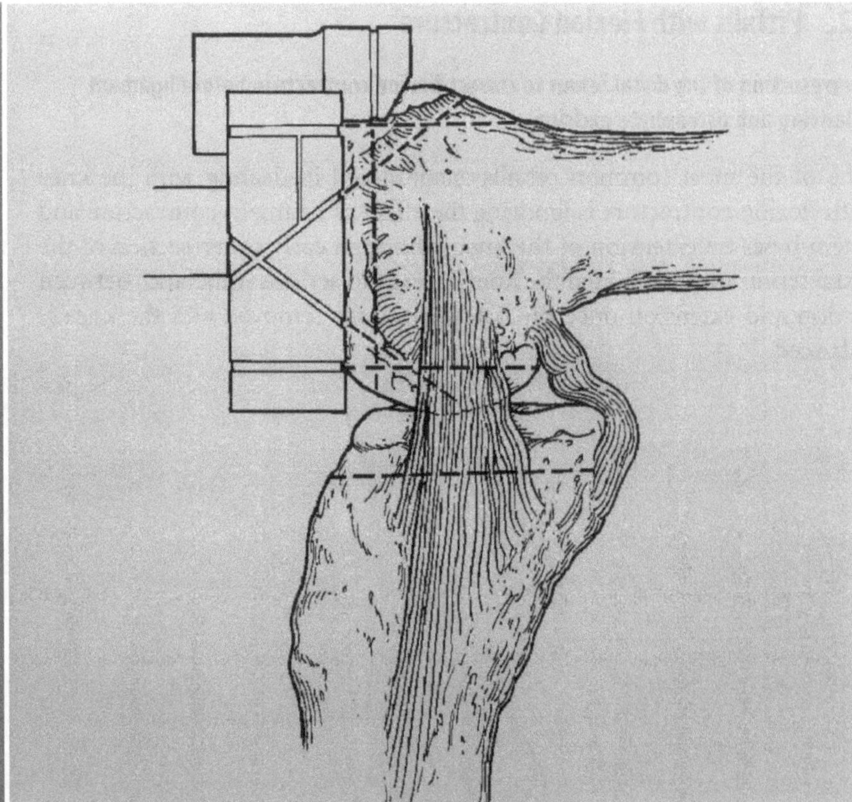

Fig. 183. Now the surfaces are removed in standard fashion, removing the thickness of implants from all surfaces.

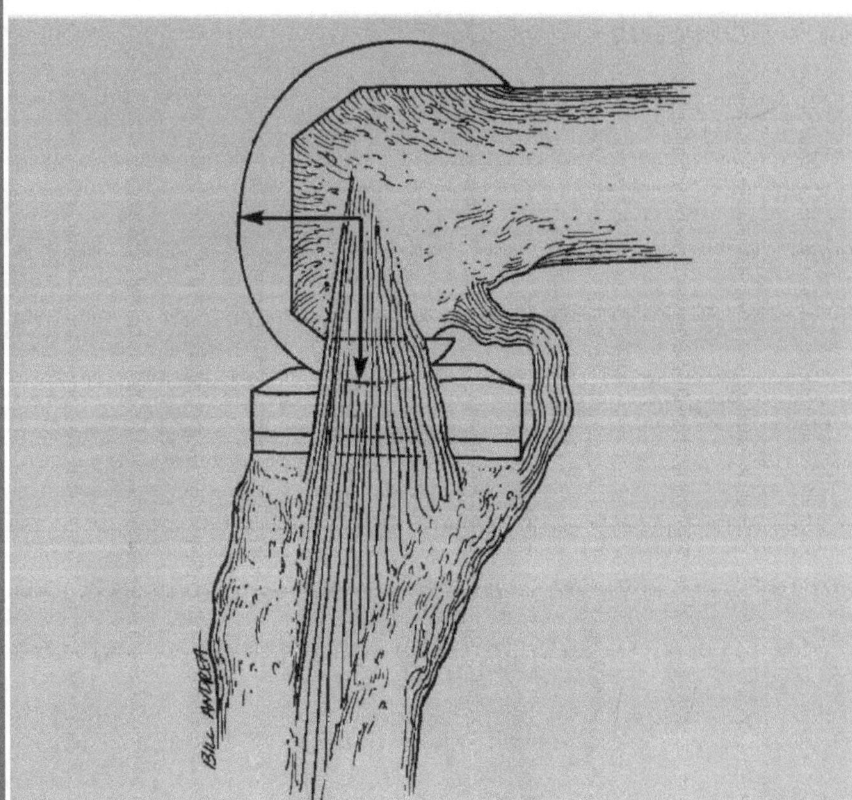

Fig. 184. The osteophytes have been removed and the implants have been inserted. The joint surface is shifted proximally, but this does not affect ligament balance in flexion.

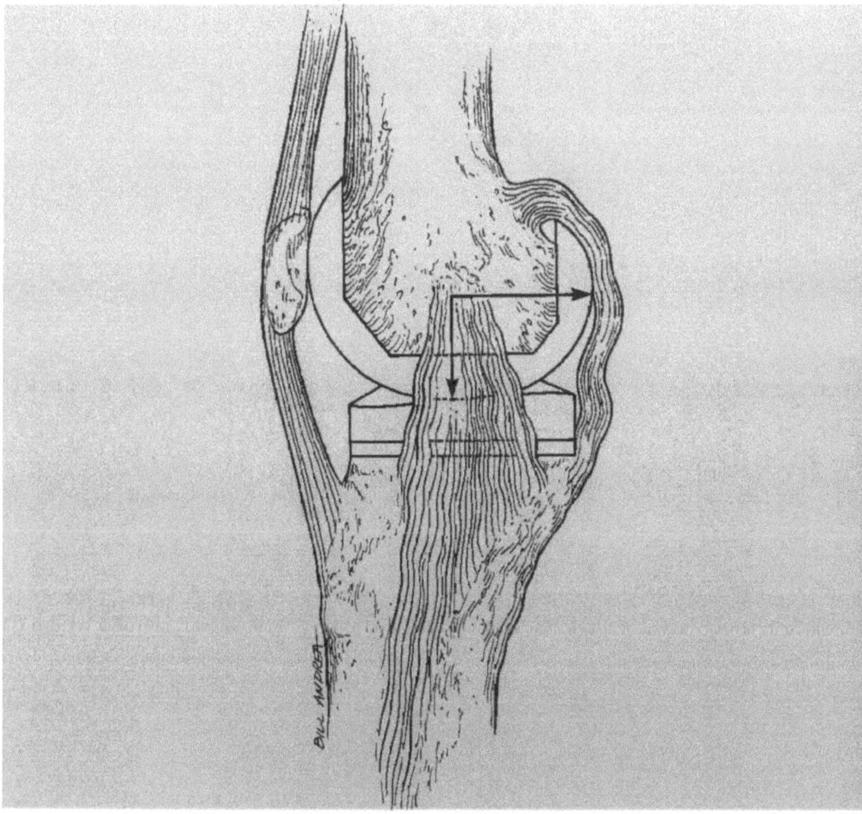

Fig. 185. The osteophytes were the major cause of flexion contracture, but they have been removed. Excessive bone has been removed from the distal surface of the femur. The knee is loose in extension, and requires a thicker spacer on the tibia.

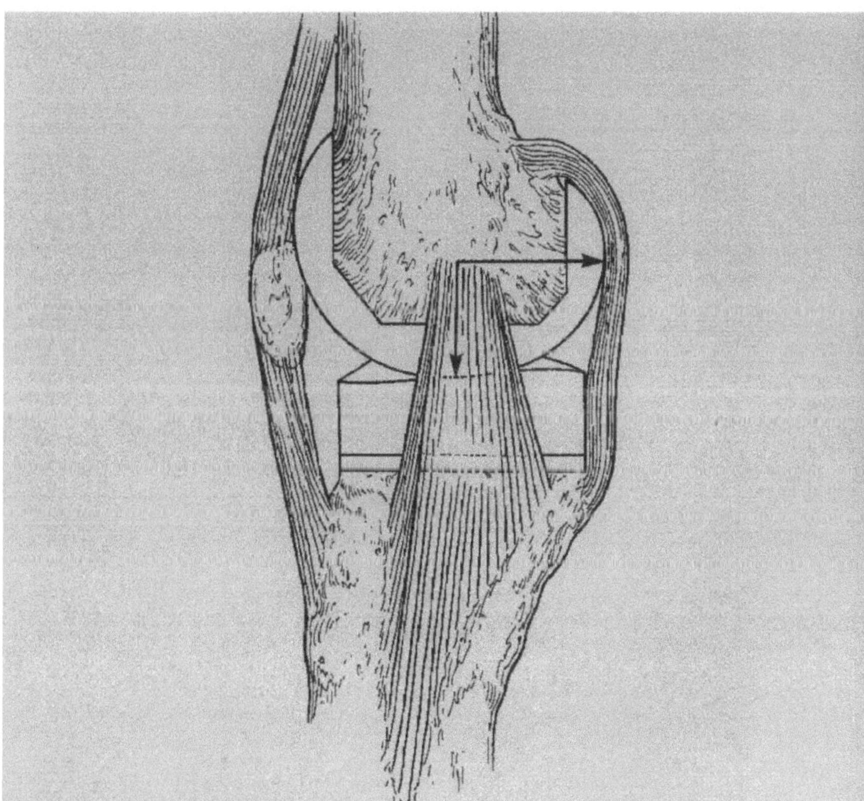

Fig. 186. Additional thickness has been added to the tibial component to stabilize the knee in extension. This raises the joint surface relative to the patella.

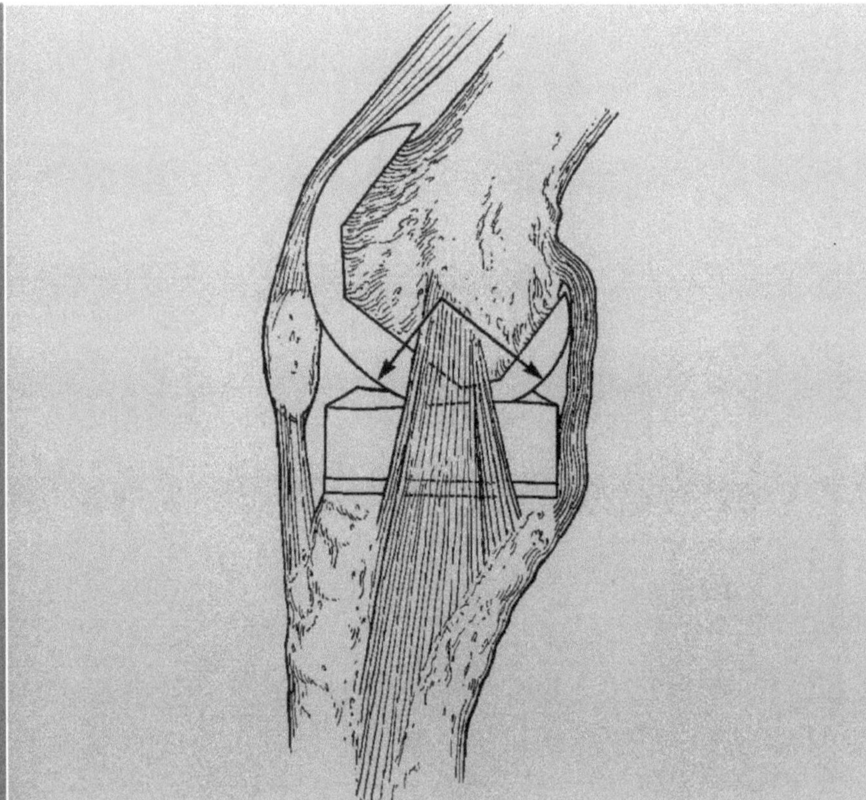

Fig. 187. With the extra thickness on the tibial component, the knee will not flex. Also, the patella may impinge on the polyethylene component.

Recurvatum

7. Recurvatum

Basic Principles

Recurvatum of the knee without major medial-lateral laxity is unusual, but when present, can be difficult to manage if the bone is not resected correctly. If the knee has global laxity along with recurvatum, this can be readily treated with a thicker tibial component, which tightens the knee through the entire flexion-extension arc. In situations with recurvatum and excessive laxity only in extension, the knee can be considered to have a loose extension space and tight flexion space. Adjustments in initial bone resection are done to correct these conditions. This entails a slightly undersized femoral component placed more distally than usual on the femur, and a posteriorly sloped tibial surface. This combination of procedures tightens the extension space and loosens the flexion space.

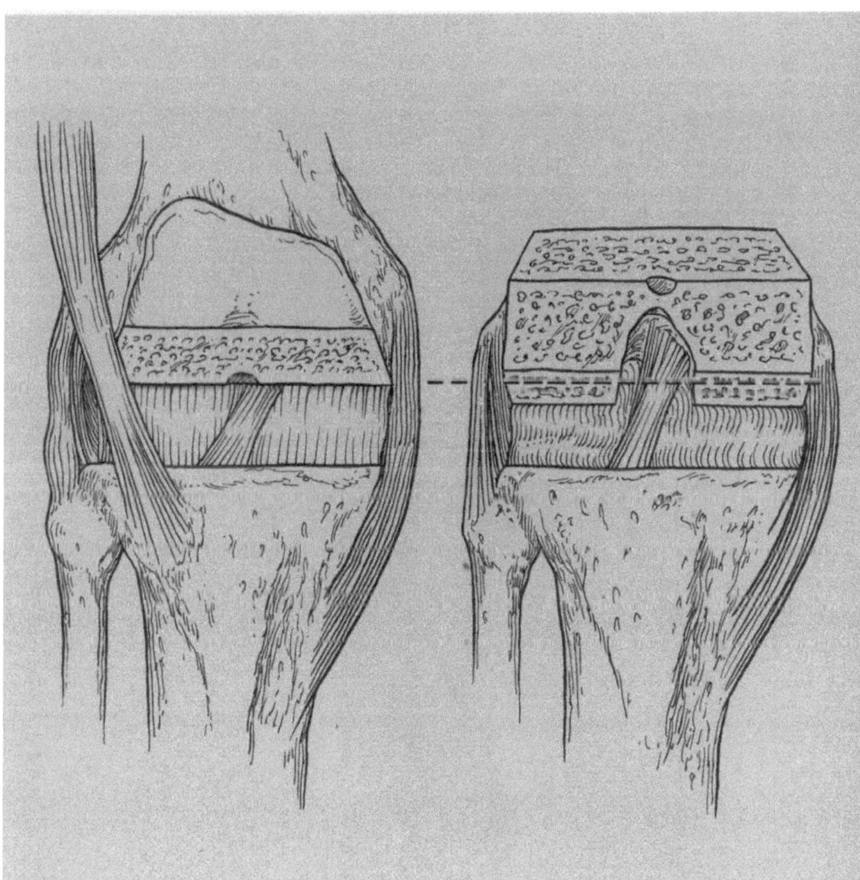

Fig. 188. In the knee with recurvatum, if the usual matched resection is done, there is an excessively large extension space and a small flexion space. After resection of normal amounts of bone, the extension space is lax (left). The flexion space is tight (right).

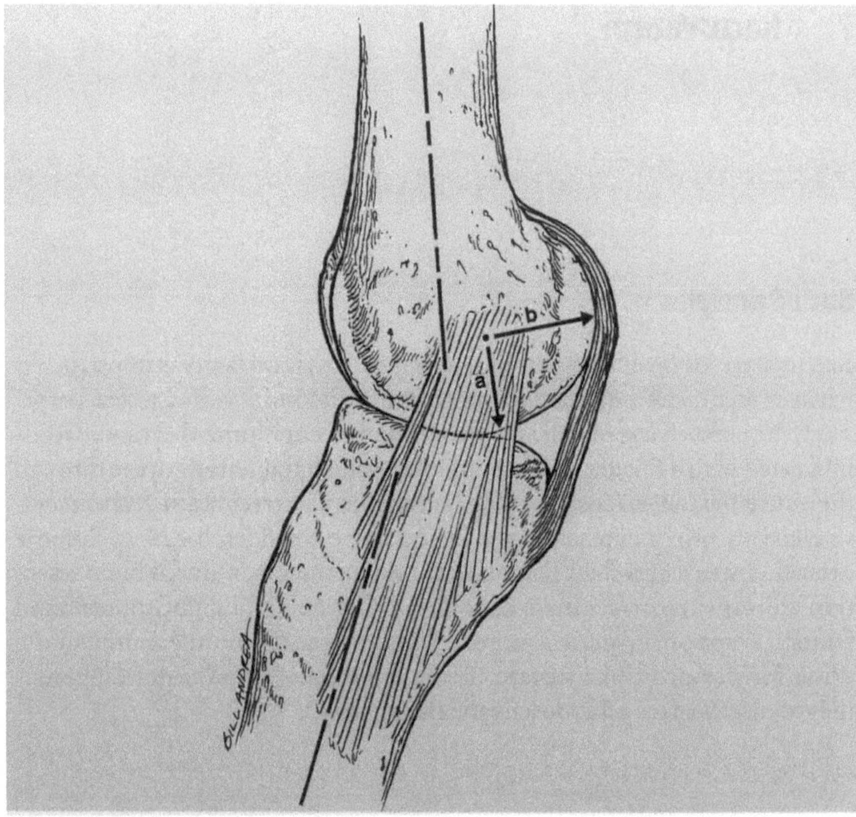

Fig. 189. As illustrated here, the collateral ligaments are competent, but the distal femoral distance (a), from the ligament attachments to the joint surface is too short, allowing the tibia to pass the midline into hyperextension before the collateral ligaments and posterior capsule are tightened.

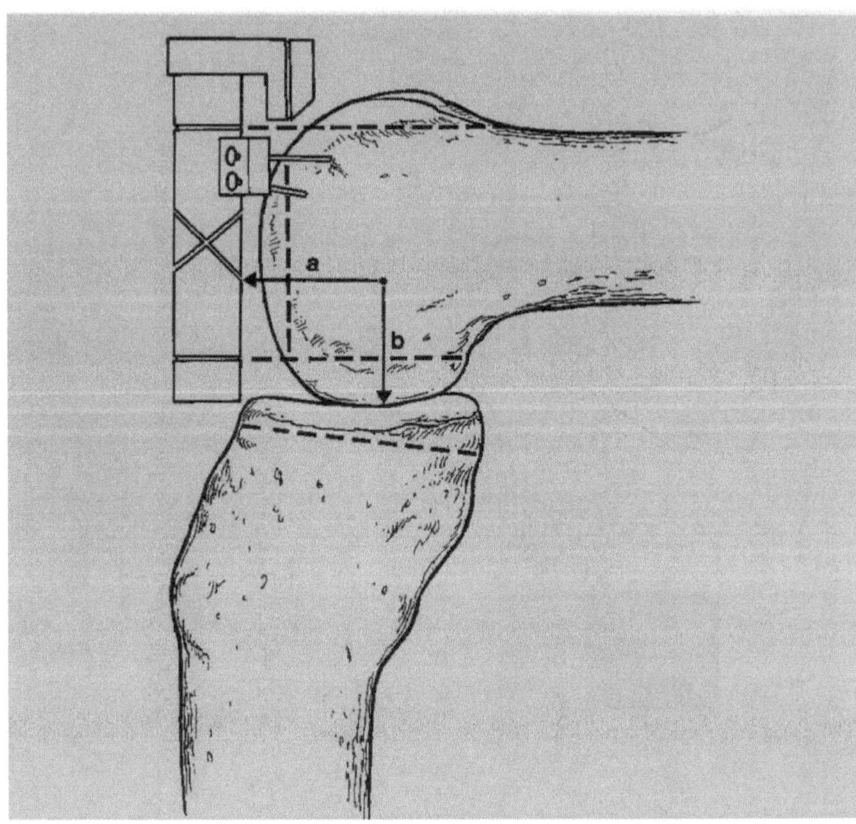

Fig. 190. The bone abnormality is corrected by underresecting the distal surface of the femur, overresecting the posterior surfaces of the femur, and sloping the tibia posteriorly. This can be achieved by applying the femoral cutting guide distal to its usual position, so that less than the thickness of the femoral component is resected. The femoral component is undersized to enlarge the flexion space. The tibial surface is sloped posteriorly to enlarge the flexion space and narrow the extension space. Now the distance a and b are more nearly equal, and the knee will be stable though the entire arc of flexion.

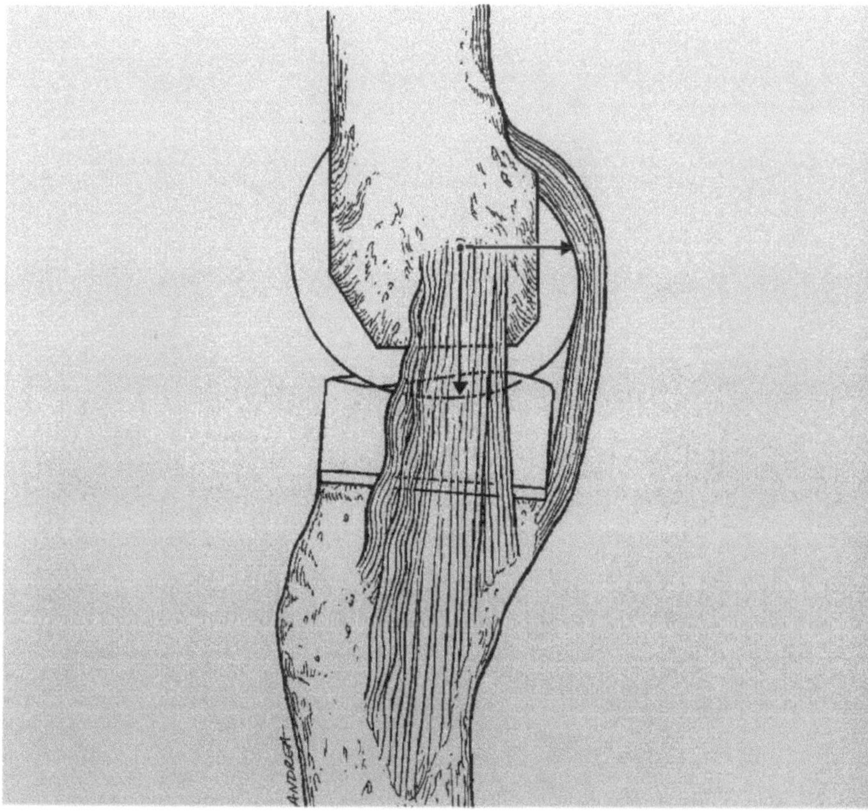

Fig. 191. The femoral component is undersized front-to-back, and placed farther distally on the femur than normally is done. Because the posterior femur was overresected, a thicker tibial spacer can be used. This also augments stability in extension. Now the posterior capsule and posterior portion of the collateral ligaments are tensioned normally in extension.

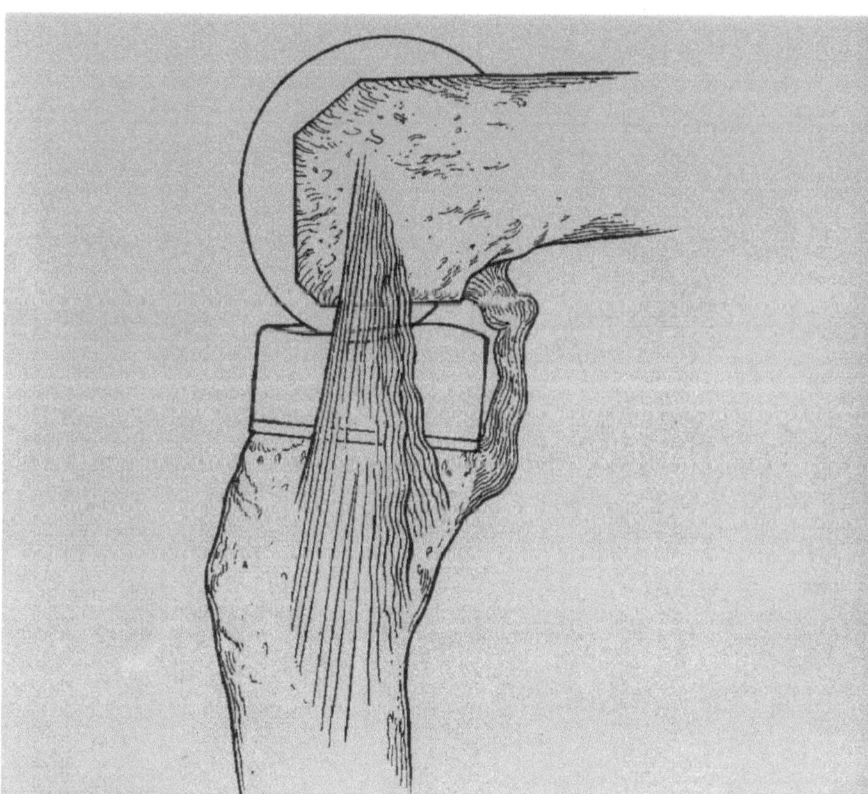

Fig. 192. In flexion the thicker tibial component affords correct ligament tensioning to fill the space that is opened by choosing a smaller femoral component. To allow deep flexion the proximal edge of the posterior femoral flange surface should be resected so that the posterior edge of the tibial polyethylene component can enter the posterior recess.

8. Summary

The structure of the knee is complex and its behavior can be unpredictable even in the most experienced hands. However, the task of replacing the bone surfaces and balancing the ligaments can be made manageable by following a logical plan based on correct alignment throughout the arc of flexion, and ligament release based on function of each ligament. Optimal knee function requires correct varus-valgus alignment in all positions of flexion. This requires reliable anatomic landmarks for alignment both in flexion and extension. The long axes of the femur and tibia and the anterior-posterior axis of the femur are highly reliable, and provide the guidelines for establishing stable alignment of the joint surfaces by placing the tibia and patellar groove correctly in the median anterior-posterior plane through the entire arc of flexion. Ligaments perform specific functions, and these functions differ in different positions of knee flexion. Knowing their function and testing their tension provides the information necessary to release only the ligaments that are excessively tight, leaving those that are performing normally. Fractional release does not destabilize the knee because other ligaments are retained, and because the peripheral attachments of the ligament to other soft tissue structures such as the periosteum or synovial-capsular tissue allow the released ligament to continue to function. Ligament release does not cause instability. Failure to align the knee and release the tight ligaments, however, does cause instability, unreliable function, and excessive wear. This manual provides an outline of how knee kinematics should be assessed and ligaments balanced in total knee arthroplasty. Although it provides specific examples of common situations encountered by the surgeon, there are thousands of scenarios that occur during this operation, so this manual should be viewed as a guide that provides the basic knowledge of how the knee functions. With this knowledge, good instruments, and sound implants, the surgeon can align, balance, and stabilize the knee even in the face of severe bone destruction and ligament contracture.

Leo A. Whiteside M.D.

MIX
Papier aus verantwortungsvollen Quellen
Paper from responsible sources
FSC® C105338

If you have any concerns about our products,
you can contact us on
ProductSafety@springernature.com

In case Publisher is established outside the EU,
the EU authorized representative is:
Springer Nature Customer Service Center GmbH
Europaplatz 3, 69115 Heidelberg, Germany

Printed by Libri Plureos GmbH
in Hamburg, Germany